Artificial Intelligence in Anesthesiology

Ming Xia • Hong Jiang
Editors

Artificial Intelligence in Anesthesiology

Springer

Editors
Ming Xia
Department of Anesthesiology
Shanghai Ninth People's Hospital,
Shanghai Jiao Tong University School
of Medicine
Shanghai, China

Hong Jiang
Department of Anesthesiology
Shanghai Ninth People's Hospital,
Shanghai Jiao Tong University School
of Medicine
Shanghai, China

ISBN 978-981-99-5924-2 ISBN 978-981-99-5925-9 (eBook)
https://doi.org/10.1007/978-981-99-5925-9

This Springer imprint is published by the registered company Springer Nature Singapore Pte Ltd.
The registered company address is: 152 Beach Road, #21-01/04 Gateway East, Singapore 189721, Singapore

Paper in this product is recyclable.

Contents

Editors and Contributors

Editors

Hong Jiang Department of Anesthesiology, Shanghai Ninth People's Hospital, Shanghai Jiao Tong University School of Medicine, Shanghai, China

Ming Xia Department of Anesthesiology, Shanghai Ninth People's Hospital, Shanghai Jiao Tong University School of Medicine, Shanghai, China

Associate Editor

Bifa Fan Department of Pain Medicine, China-Japan Friendship Hospital, Beijing, China

Contributors

Shuang Cao Department of Anesthesiology, Shanghai Ninth People's Hospital, Shanghai Jiao Tong University School of Medicine, Shanghai, China

Ningning Ji Department of Anesthesiology, Shanghai Ninth People's Hospital, Shanghai Jiao Tong University School of Medicine, Shanghai, China

Chenyu Jin Department of Anesthesiology, Shanghai Ninth People's Hospital, Shanghai Jiao Tong University School of Medicine, Shanghai, China

Bei Pei Department of Anesthesiology, Shanghai Ninth People's Hospital, Shanghai Jiao Tong University School of Medicine, Shanghai, China

Artificial Intelligence: An Overview

Hong Jiang

The development of artificial intelligence (AI) has a short history, starting in the 1950s, yet after continuous iterations and upgrades, today, it can be said to have penetrated all areas of society, especially people's lifestyles have also undergone radical changes. Clothing, food, housing, and transportation, while pursuing efficiency, people are also in pursuit of a more personalized and comfortable experience, which is also reflected in seeking medical care. Therefore, experts and scholars in the medical field are rooted in their own professions and actively seek cross-disciplinary cooperation to promote the beautiful vision of intelligent and smart medical care to become a reality.

1 History of Artificial Intelligence in Medicine

The origin of AI can be traced back to Alan Turing, who first described the concept of using computers to simulate intelligent behavior and critical thinking in 1950 (Ramesh et al. 2004). He introduced a test named after him as "Turing test," to clarify if computers were able to master human intelligence (Greenhill 2020). In 1956, John McCarthy proposed the concept of artificial intelligence (Puppe 1997).

The early stage of AI, which was from the 1950s to 1970s, bred machines that were capable of making inferences or decisions like human intelligence (Kaul et al. 2020). The first industrial robot arm (Unimate; Unimation, Danbury, Conn, USA) was added to the General Motors assembly line in 1961 to automate die casting (Moran 2007). Unimate can perform actions following exact commands. Three years later, Eliza was developed and it was a prototype of future AI that could make a communication like humans by employing pattern matching and substitution methodology (Weizenbaum 1966). In 1966, Shakey, the "first electronic person," created by the Stanford Research Institute, was introduced. As the first mobile robot capable of interpreting instructions, it no longer simply followed a step-by-step instruction and acted, but was able to process more complex instructions and perform appropriate actions (Kuipers et al. 2017). This was an important milestone in robotics and artificial intelligence.

After decades of advancement, AI now consists of computer algorithms that can mimic the characteristics of human intelligence, and its success is due to the tremendous growth in computing ability and data availability. Over the past decade, AI applications based on machine learning (ML), deep learning (DL), and neural net-

H. Jiang (✉)
Department of Anesthesiology, Shanghai Ninth People's Hospital, Shanghai Jiao Tong University School of Medicine, Shanghai, China

M. Xia, H. Jiang (eds.), *Artificial Intelligence in Anesthesiology*,
https://doi.org/10.1007/978-981-99-5925-9_1

work algorithms have made significant breakthroughs in areas such as computer vision (CV), intelligent robotics, natural language understanding, semantic recognition, and image processing.

However, the combination of AI with medicine began very slowly. Starting from the 1970s, AI methods were applied in the medical field to improve the efficiency of disease diagnosis and treatment, which led to the emergence of artificial intelligence in medicine (AIM). One of the first prototypes demonstrating the feasibility of applying AI to medicine was the development of a consultation program for glaucoma using the CASNET model, a cause-and-effect correlation network consisting of three separate programs: model building, consultation, and a database built and maintained by collaborators. The model allowed for the application of disease-specific information to individual patients and provided advice to physicians on patient management. It was developed in 1976 (Weiss et al. 1978). Developed in the early 1970s, MYCIN is a "backward-chaining" artificial intelligence system (Shortliffe et al. 1975). Based on physician input of patient information and a knowledge base of approximately 600 rules, MYCIN could provide a list of potential bacterial pathogens and then suggest appropriate adjustments to antibiotic regimens based on the patient's weight. MYCIN became the framework for the later rule-based system EMYCIN. Later, INTERNIST-1 used the same framework as EMYCIN and a larger medical knowledge base to assist primary care physicians with diagnosis (Kulikowski 2019).

In 1986, the University of Massachusetts released DXplain, a decision support system that generates a differential diagnosis by entering a patient's symptoms (Amisha et al. 2019). It is also an electronic medical textbook that provides detailed descriptions of diseases and other reference material. At the time of its first release, DXplain was able to provide information on about 500 diseases and was subsequently expanded to over 2400 diseases (The Massachusetts General Hospital Laboratory of Computer Science 2023). By the late 1990s, there was a renewed interest in ML, particularly in the medical community, which, along with the technological developments described above, set the stage for the modern era of AIM.

In the last two decades, AIM has changed profoundly. In 2007, IBM created an open-domain question-answering system called Watson, which competed against human participants and won first place on the 2011 television game show Jeopardy! The technology, called DeepQA, uses natural language processing and various searches to analyze data on unstructured content to generate possible answers compared to traditional systems that use forward reasoning (rules from data to conclusions), backward reasoning (rules from conclusions to data) or hand-crafted if-then rules (Ferrucci et al. 2013). This system is easier to use, easier to maintain, and more cost-effective. By extracting information from patients' electronic medical records and other electronic resources, one can apply DeepQA technology to provide evidence-based medical responses. Thus, it offers new possibilities for evidence-based clinical decision-making (Ferrucci et al. 2013; Mintz and Brodie 2019). In 2017, Bakkar et al. (2018) successfully identified novel RNA-binding proteins altered in amyotrophic lateral sclerosis using IBM Watson.

Given this momentum, AIM began to evolve rapidly along with improvements in computer hardware and software programs that made digital medicine more accessible. Natural language processing transforms chatbots from superficial communication (Eliza) to meaningful conversational interfaces. This technology was applied to Apple's virtual assistant Siri in 2011 and to Amazon's virtual assistant Alexa in 2014. Pharmabot is a chatbot developed in 2015 to assist in medication education for pediatric patients and their parents, and Mandy was created in 2017 as an automated patient intake for a primary care clinic program (Comendador et al. 2015; Ni et al. 2017). Deep learning (DL) marks an important advance in AIM. In contrast to machine learning (ML), which uses a set number of features and requires human input, DL can be trained to classify data on its own. Although DL was first studied in the 1950s, its use in medicine was limited by the "overfitting" problem. Overfitting occurs when ML is too focused on a specific dataset and cannot accurately process new datasets, which can be the result of insufficient computational power and a lack of training data. These limitations were overcome in the 2000s with the advent of larger datasets and significant increases in computational power.

A convolutional neural network (CNN) is a DL algorithm applied to image processing that simulates the behavior of interconnected neurons in the human brain. A CNN is composed of several layers that analyze the input image to identify patterns and create specific filters. The final result is a combination of all the features of the fully connected layers (Hoogenboom et al. 2020; Yang and Bang 2019). Several CNN algorithms are now available, including Le-NET, AlexNet, VGG, GoogLeNet, and ResNet (Vinsard et al. 2019). The advent of ML and DL expanded the use of AIM, creating opportunities for personalized medicine instead of algorithm-based medicine alone. Predictive models can be used for diagnosis of diseases, prediction of treatment response, and possibly future preventive medicine. AI may improve the accuracy of diagnosis, increase the efficiency of workflow and clinical operations, facilitate better disease and treatment monitoring, and improve the accuracy of surgery and overall patient outcomes (Kaul et al. 2020; Yazhou et al. 2022).

2 Common Technologies of AIM

The development of AI has emerged in two main historical directions: symbolism and connectionism. The expert system (ES), which became popular in the 1980s, was a classic example of symbolism. Since the 1990s, connectionist-based learning approaches have emerged, with the advantage that data, rather than human experts, provided the assurance of accuracy (Su 1994).

2.1 Machine Learning (ML)

The concept of ML was introduced by Samuel in 1959 and can be expressed as the ability of data to be learned by a computer without explicit programming (Sameul 1959). Quinlan (1988) proposed the decision tree (DT) algorithm, which can classify data based on established rules (Quinlan 1988). Vladimir proposed support vector machines (SVM), which is a widely used supervised ML algorithm, commonly used in classification and regression problems (Huang et al. 2018). HO (1998) proposed the random forest (RF) algorithm, which can effectively complete feature extraction.

In recent years, ML has been increasingly used in the medical field, aiming to help physicians predict disease and prognosis outcomes. ML has reached important milestones in its development, achieving similar or better accuracy than human experts. Typical supervised tasks include regression and classification, unsupervised tasks include dimensionality reduction, clustering, and outlier detection, while semi-supervised learning is a hybrid framework between supervised and unsupervised, with applications such as segmentation or classification of images using partially labeled data (Burton 2nd et al. 2020).

There are still significant gaps and room for improvement in ML technology. Clinicians want to understand the scientific basis for clinical decisions so that they can make independent judgments about effectiveness and ensure that they are appropriate for all types of patients. However, clinicians do not have intuitive access to the underlying mechanisms in ML technology to understand how to make specific recommendations for a given clinical situation, which is often referred to as a "black box" problem. Especially when clinicians' prior experience conflicts with the recommendations of AI methods, physicians often lack trust in AI methods, and advances in "interpretable AI" may address this issue in the future.

2.2 Deep Learning (DL)

Since the 1990s, ML methods have evolved and been improved, giving birth to what is now popularly known as DL. DL was a subset of ML algorithms and was first introduced by Aizenberg and Hinton et al. in the early twenty-first century (Schmidhuber 2015). It was called "deep" because it was organized in layers at multiple levels and could automatically extract meaningful features from big data. AI has been proposed to improve the accuracy, consistency, and efficiency of medical imaging reports. Arterys became the first cloud-based DL application in healthcare approved by the FDA in 2017. Arterys' first product, CardioAI, was able to analyze cardiac MRI images in seconds, providing information such as cardiac ejection fraction. This application has since expanded to include liver and lung imaging, chest and musculoskeletal X-ray images, and non-contrast head CT images.

Currently, the application of DL in medical images has achieved great progress, but it still has certain limitations. First, medical datasets bear the characteristics of unevenness and are often single-centered with small sample sizes, but DL relies strongly on high-quality large datasets, which may bring expensive economic costs. Second, DL models have a large number of learning parameters and a risk of overfitting, so they lack stability and repeatability in applications. Finally, similar to ML technology, DL also has the disadvantage of "black box," which causes suspicion in both doctors and patients while applying it in the clinical setting. Therefore, DL technology should be applied in appropriate medical fields to improve the accuracy of diagnosis and treatment.

2.3 Expert System

ES is a computer system that simulates the decision-making ability of human experts, which can reason and solve a series of complex problems using the existing knowledge system, and is one of the early successful AI software (Urrea and Mignogna 2020). The development phase of ES can be roughly divided into three stages: the initiation period (1965–1971), the development period (1972–1977), and the maturity period (1978–present). Currently, ES has demonstrated strong clinical decision-making ability and has greater advantages in disease screening and diagnosis. However, ES is more dependent on human experts, who may make mistakes or have subjective tendencies. The subsequent application still needs to integrate the clinical experience of physicians and patient history to improve the accuracy of the system. In addition, the application of ES requires continuous updating of medical knowledge and findings to provide clinicians with cutting-edge diagnoses and treatment plans.

2.4 Intelligent Robots

In 1979, the American Institute of Robotics introduced the concept of Intelligent Robots (IR), which is defined as a reprogrammable multifunctional manipulator designed to perform tasks using a variety of programmed materials, components, and tools (Beasley 2012). Since the 1980s, IR has been gradually used in surgical procedures. Currently, FDA-approved robotic surgical systems include ZUES, Da Vinci, and automated endoscopic systems. With the advantages of being minimally invasive, precise, and intelligent, IR has been widely used in many fields such as orthopedics, gynecology, urology, and dentistry.

Whereas, IR used in clinical practice were often discrete robots with limited mobility. In recent years, continuous robots have been proposed as a new type of bionic robot with a flexible structure of "invertebrates," which has flexible bending characteristics and good environmental adaptability and is expected to gradually replace discrete robots as the main force of future surgical procedures (Gao et al. 2020). However, IR still has the disadvantages of high cost, large size, and limited application scope.

3 Healthcare Applications of AI

The combination of AI and healthcare focuses on the datasets. By collecting and analyzing tremendous amount of patient data, AI can help doctors and patients screen, diagnose, and predict risk factors and diseases.

3.1 AI in Medical Imaging and Diagnostics

At present, AIM technology has been applied in the screening of many kinds of malignant tumors, which can automatically screen the benign and malignant nature of cancerous areas, such as the screening for digestive tumors and breast cancer. AI also improved the assessment in medical imaging to detect diabetic retinopathy and achieved high specificity and sensitivity (Yazhou et al. 2022). In addition, the diagnostic role of AI has been emerging. Studies have been conducted to testify the sensitivity, accuracy, and AUC value of AIM technologies, the results of which showed that they accomplished good automation performance (Yazhou et al. 2022). Diseases that AIM technologies can well diagnose include infectious diseases, medical diseases, and surgical diseases.

However, it should be noticed that the accuracy of AI screening models has a significant impact on physicians' clinical decisions, and when models are inaccurate in their predictions, their effectiveness in aiding screening is often substantially reduced. In addition, the lower prevalence of certain diseases and smaller sample sizes make false positives more likely. Given these shortcomings, the use of AI models in the clinic continues to face significant challenges, and the potential shortcomings of model-assisted screening should be considered in the development and application of AI tools.

3.2 AI in Risk Prediction

AIM enables automatic assessment and early warning of risks and provides effective clinical decision support. AI-based approaches to early warning systems have been proposed and implemented in predicting infection, chronic disease, and treatment risks. However, their implementation aroused disparate opinions among clinicians due to the nontransparency and uncertainty of AI technologies such as ML, DL, and so on.

3.3 AI as Assistive Therapy Tools

Currently, a variety of decision support tools based on AI approaches have performed excellently as experts in making a judgment on diseases. Their application effectively improved empirical treatment decisions, shortened treatment time, and lowered costs. These tools included therapeutic decision support, drug development and management, and robot-assisted surgery. First, the application of therapeutic decision support included the use of ML models to determine the threshold dose of radiotherapy that different organs can receive when administering radiation therapy to oncology patients, thereby delineating the organs at risk and providing guidance for the treatment. Secondly, prescription drugs are critical to the treatment of diseases and the safety of patients' lives. Prescription errors may trigger high morbidity and medical burden. ML-based prescription recognition and decision system can automatically warn of prescription errors and correct them, which can improve the existing prescription error warning system and enhance the efficiency of medication management. Besides, robotic surgery has been widely used in orthopedics, biliary, pharyngeal, and liver surgeries, and achieved good surgical results and prognosis, possessing the prospect of expanding applications in other departments.

Yet, most of the current adjuvant tools target specific diseases, and their generalized value needs to be further explored; therefore, increasing the diversity of cases, collecting long-term follow-up and post-follow-up data, and developing multicenter and multisite planning systems can provide better clinical treatment guidance.

4 Applications of AI in Anesthesiology

In recent years, AI has flourished in the medical field, improving the efficiency of healthcare professionals. As an important discipline of clinical medicine, the development of anesthesiology is crucial to the progress of the medical field. In daily anesthesia work, due to the variability of surgical operations, individual patient differences, and the unpredictability of clinical events, anesthesiologists must respond to a large number of clinical events simultaneously and accurately, and thus may suffer from mental exhaustion and consequently adverse outcomes under prolonged high-pressure environments. To address this prominent problem, while improving anesthesia efficiency and safeguarding patient safety in the perioperative period, AI has been applied to clinical anesthesiology, and a variety of intelligent anesthesia systems have been developed, and clinical anesthesia is evolving toward automated anesthesia. This section will briefly introduce how AI intersects with anesthesiology.

4.1 Ultrasound-Guided Anesthesia

Ultrasound has become a major diagnostic and operational tool for anesthesiologists. Nerve blocks, intraoperative echocardiographic monitoring, and difficult arteriovenous cannulation all require ultrasound assistance. Accurate recognition of ultrasound images is the foundation for anesthesiologists to master ultrasound technology. The accurate recognition of medical images can be effectively improved by using the AI deep learning algorithm CNN, the full name of which is a convolutional neural network, and its operation mode is similar to the human eye perceiving the outside world. Firstly, the local receptive fields are obtained by disassembling the image layer by layer, and then the RBG values of individual pixel points within each receptive field are calculated, and then the information of each local receptive field is integrated to recognize the content of the whole image. With the continuous innovation of the operating function and the speed of operation, CNN can perform image recognition quickly and accurately, and the effect can be comparable to that of human eyes. The use of echocardiography, ultrasound-guided nerve blocks, and subarachnoid blocks can greatly improve the efficiency of anesthesia and guarantee anesthesia and surgical safety. Details will be illustrated in detail in subsequent chapters.

4.2 Anesthesia Monitoring

One of the main responsibilities of anesthesiologists is to monitor patients' vital signs during anesthesia and to ensure patients' life safety, a process also called anesthesia monitoring. During surgery, it is necessary to avoid both too shallow or too deep anesthesia. The former may induce intraoperative awareness, while the latter may affect the patient's transition, both of which can cause damage to the patient's physiology and psychology. The degree of stress at different stages of surgery varies, so it is necessary to constantly adapt the depth of anesthesia to the surgical stimulation. Therefore, each anesthesia and surgery is like a huge project. Dumont et al. described anesthesia control systems, including feedforward and feedback systems as well as multiple examples of different closed-loops (Dumont and Ansermino 2013). Li et al. (2020) combined LSTM with a fuzzy autocoder to predict the depth of anesthesia according to EEG during anesthesia. Compared with other traditional prediction models, this model had the highest prediction accuracy of 85.56%. With this model, the occurrence of postoperative complications induced by too-deep anesthesia can be decreased and intraoperative awareness can be avoided. Therefore, it was expected to be promoted in clinical applications.

4.3 Anesthesia Event Prediction

For perioperative care risk prediction, various techniques in machine learning, neural networks, and fuzzy logic have been applied. For instance, neural networks were used to predict the hypnotic effect of propofol induction dose (measured by BIS) (sensitivity of 82.35%, specificity of 64.38%, area under the curve of 0.755) and were found to exceed the average estimate of practicing anesthesiologists (sensitivity of 20.64%, specificity of 92.51%, area under the curve of 0.5605) (Lin et al. 2002). Neural networks were also used to predict recovery rates from neuromuscular blockade and episodes of hypotension after induction or during spinal anesthesia, while other machine learning methods have been tested to automatically classify preoperative patient acuity, namely ASA status, define difficult laryngoscopy findings, identify respiratory depression during conscious sedation, and to help to decide the best anesthetic approach for pediatric surgery (Hashimoto et al. 2020).

Machine learning approaches used in critical care were not limited to large database studies. In a single-center randomized controlled trial that compared a machine learning alert system using six vital sign parameters as features with an electronic health record-based alert system using other criteria for predicting sepsis, the machine learning alert system outperformed the Systemic Inflammatory Response Syndrome criteria, the Sequential Organ Failure Assessment Score, and the Rapid Sequential Organ Failure Assessment Score in detecting sepsis. With this alert system, the average length of stay was reduced by 20.6%, and in-hospital mortality was reduced by 58% (Shimabukuro et al. 2017).

4.4 Pain Management

Pain management is also an important responsibility of anesthesiologists. Pain is an inevitable experience during surgery, but the combination of multiple anesthetics often masks the typical manifestations of pain, preventing anesthesiologists from detecting inadequate analgesia in a timely manner and causing serious physical and psychological trauma to patients. Kharghanian et al. (2016) used a convolutional deep confidence network for recognizing facial expression features, by which whether pain presented was determined, and results obtained had an accuracy of 95%, which can reduce the incidence of pain that failed to diagnose. Lim et al. (2019) constructed a deep learning model for intraoperative pain assessment and imported the data of heart rate and its variability collected intraoperatively into three algorithms: deep belief network (DBN), multilayer perceptron, and support vector machine. The accuracy of these three prediction models was evaluated by the AUC area under the ROC curve, and the results showed that DBN had the highest accuracy, which was 84.1%. This model may serve as a basis of a pain assessment system for surgical patients in the future to prevent inadequate intraoperative analgesia. Rodriguez et al. (2017) developed a CNN + LSTM model for guiding the development of postoperative analgesia protocols. The composite model first extracted facial features from images using the CNN algorithm, and then trained LSTM algorithm with these facial feature data for pain grading, with an accuracy of 97.2% for estimating pain levels. The application of these AI technologies to accurately identify and assess pain set a foundation for realizing the concept of "pain-free treatment."

4.5 Airway Management

Airway management is an indispensable skill mastered by all anesthesiologists. Throughout the entire process of anesthesia and surgery, ranging from preoperative airway assessment to postoperative airway management in the SICU, a secure and current airway guarantees the safety of patients and surgery. With the assistance of AI technologies, airway management became more scientific and effective, especially in the case of difficult airways. Related techniques include face recognition analysis, speech feature analysis, and support vector machines. An AI model for difficult intubation classification using CNN was described in the study by Hayasaka et al. for rapid identification and management of difficult intubations in emergency situations (Hayasaka et al. 2021). The chief editors of this book and their team are also dedicated to clinical research related to the application of AI in managing difficult airway.

4.6 Clinical Decision Support System

Anesthesia records are a major component of clinical anesthesia, and patients' perioperative data can provide a reference for subsequent anesthesia management and case management. The current anesthesia information management systems (AIMS) in major hospitals can collect data from sources such as monitors, hospital information systems, ventilators, and anesthesia workstations in real time. At the same time, anesthesiologists record the patient's fluid balance status, surgery, medication, special events, and other information in real time according to intraoperative anesthesia management. In a word, the anesthesia record is a comprehensive database of real-time information during the patient's surgery.

Clinical Decision Support System (CDSS) is a hardware system that provides real-time decision aid for anesthesiologists. The system mainly collects data from AIMS and categorizes them by transforming, filtering, and filling in the missing data, etc. into useful and other types of data. The decision processor applies algorithms to process the data and determines whether to make notifications or alerts on the AIMS according to the set decision rules. Anesthesiologists, thus, make decisions on the following treatments according to the notifications.

4.7 Clinical Skill Training and Assessment

AI is changing various aspects of clinical skill training and assessment in anesthesiology. On one hand, technologies such as "real-time collection and identification of multi-source clinical teaching data," "analysis of teaching indicators for artificial intelligence methods and construction of prediction and warning model," "teaching evaluation algorithm and intelligent teaching intervention hint" can track and analyze students' performance and provide advises for improvement automatically. On the other hand, against the background of the COVID-19 pandemic, activities of all kinds are somehow halted and may be suspended at any time. Using AI to score student performance on both written and in-person components of clinical skills assessment is promising and efficient. Researchers showed their confidence in the positive future of the application of AI expert systems in students' training, anesthesia teaching, and hospital development.

5 Challenges to AI Adoption in Medicine and the Way Forward

5.1 Limitations and Challenges

5.1.1 Role of Anesthesiologists

The role of the anesthesiologist has been challenged. Whether automated machines will gradually replace anesthesiologists has also become a controversial issue. In recent years, various types of AI systems have emerged and are challenging human capabilities in various aspects. ChatGPT, introduced by OpenAI, has attracted a lot of attention from different communities with its outstanding intelligence and interaction capabilities. It not only participated in scientific research but also outperformed senior clinicians in disease diagnosis and treatment plan development. For example, leading international journals have published articles with it as a co-author, and journals have established publication rules for ChatGPT as more and more scholars draw on it to complete their research. In the field of anesthesia, Hemmerling (2020) suggested that robotic anesthesia should be realized in the future. Nevertheless, we believe that the adoption of automated machines should be primarily aimed at assisting clinicians with selected simple and repetitive clinical procedures, reducing workload, and allowing physicians to focus on the most important tasks. Whether AI will replace anesthesiologists in the future will depend on the state of the art. In addition, clinicians need to be aware that overreliance on machines can lead to the degradation of their clinical skills, such as their independent judgment of the clinical environment and their ability to handle emergencies may be diminished, which may pose a threat to clinical safety (Loeb and Cannesson 2017).

5.1.2 Data

The premise of machine learning processing data is to ensure the integrity and accuracy of the data, when faced with incomplete or false data, performance will be significantly reduced. Moreover, AI algorithms are also susceptible to data bias. In addition to the basic research biases that clinicians have been taught such as sampling and blinding, we must also consider implicit and explicit biases in the healthcare system that can affect the large-scale data that is or will be used to train AI. Clinical trial eligibility for specific patient populations, implicit bias in treatment decisions in real-world care, and other forms of bias can greatly affect the types of predictions that AI may make and influence clinical decisions (Murthy et al. 2004). Char et al. cited the example of withdrawing patients with traumatic brain injury from care (Char et al. 2018). AI may analyze data from the neuro ICU and interpret patterns of death following traumatic brain injury as a necessary consequence of the injury, rather than as a secondary cause of clinical decisions to withdraw life support. Therefore, it is imperative that practicing clinicians collaborate or engage in dialogue with data scientists to ensure appropriate interpretation of data analysis.

5.1.3 Ethical Implications

The black box problem is one of the disturbing concerns for users of AI. A black box result means that an algorithm can give a clinician or researcher a prediction, but cannot provide further information about why such a prediction was made. In the case of explainable AI, efforts are underway to improve the transparency of algorithms. Explainable AI aims to develop models that make it easier to explain its results such as by showing which features it may rely on to produce its predictions, with the ultimate goal of improving the transparency and winning human trust and understanding of its predictions. Some techniques in AI are easier to explain than others. For example, decision trees allow great transparency because each decision node can be reviewed and evaluated, whereas DL is currently evaluated by induction. That is, in a DL model, it may not be possible to clearly explain why each node makes certain predictions, but the model can be asked to come up with relevant features or examples from its training data of skeletal radiographs to explain why a particular prediction was made about the patient's bone age. In addition to concerns about transparency and trust in the model, AI is excellent at demonstrating correlation or identifying patterns, but it is not yet able to determine causality—at least not to the extent needed for clinical implementation (Hashimoto et al. 2020).

5.2 Future Prospects

Artificial intelligence algorithms have not outperformed humans yet; however, AI's ability to quickly and accurately sift through large amounts of data and discover correlations and patterns that are imperceptible to human cognition will make it a valuable tool for clinicians. In pathology, AI has been shown to enhance clinicians' diagnostic capabilities, for example, by reducing the error rate in identifying cancer-positive lymph nodes. This reduction in errors is due to its ability to reduce the size of histopathology sections that human pathologists must review, allowing more attention to be focused on smaller areas (Hashimoto et al. 2020). Similarly, AI technology that can help monitor anesthesia depth, maintain drug infusions, or predict intraoperative hypotension will allow practicing anesthesiologists to be more effective and efficient in providing care.

Anesthesiologists should continue to collaborate with data scientists and engineers to provide their valuable clinical insights into the development of AI to ensure that the technology is clinically applicable, i.e., that the data used to train the algorithm is valid, representative of a broad patient population, and that the interpretation of that data is clinically meaningful. Therefore, anesthesiologists should work with other healthcare providers such as surgeons, intensive care doctors, nurses, and patients to help develop strategies for the optimal use of AI. Anesthesiology has been a leader in implementing and achieving patient safety initiatives, and AI can serve as a new tool to continue innovation in the delivery of safe anesthesia care.

6 Conclusion

The core of medicine and anesthesiology is still human intervention. Although algorithms may 1 day surpass humans in integrating complex, huge, structured data sets, much of the data that clinicians collect from patients comes from positive patient–physician interactions and patients' trust in the physician. While knowledge and training for trusting AI models may be developed in the future, it remains to be seen to what extent patients are willing to trust algorithms and how patients wish to receive the results conveyed by the algorithms. Therefore, additional qualitative research is required to better understand the ethical, cultural, and social implications of incorporating AI into clinical workflows (Hashimoto et al. 2020).

References

Amisha MP, Pathania M, et al. Overview of artificial intelligence in medicine. J Family Med Prim Care. 2019;8:2328–31.

Bakkar N, Kovalik T, Lorenzini I, et al. Artificial intelligence in neurodegenerative disease research: use of IBM Watson to identify additional RNA-binding proteins altered in amyotrophic lateral sclerosis. Acta Neuropathol. 2018;135:227–47.

Beasley RA. Medical robots: current systems and research directions. J Robotics. 2012;2012:401613.

Burton W 2nd, Myers C, Rullkoetter P. Semi-supervised learning for automatic segmentation of the knee from MRI with convolutional neural networks. Comput Methods Prog Biomed. 2020;189:105328. https://doi.org/10.1016/j.cmpb.2020.105328. Epub 2020 Jan 11

Char DS, Shah NH, Magnus D. Implementing machine learning in health care - addressing ethical challenges. N Engl J Med. 2018;378:981–3.

Comendador B, Francisco B, Medenilla J, et al. Pharmabot: a pediatric generic medicine consultant chatbot. J Automat Control Eng. 2015;3:137–40.

Dumont GA, Ansermino JM. Closed-loop control of anesthesia: a primer for anesthesiologists. Anesth Analg. 2013;117:1130–8.

Ferrucci DL, Bagchi S, Gondek D, et al. Watson: beyond jeopardy! Artif Intell. 2013;199-200:93–105.

Gao Y, Takagi K, Kato T, Shono N, Hata N. Continuum robot with follow-the-leader motion for endoscopic third ventriculostomy and tumor biopsy. IEEE Trans Biomed Eng. 2020;67(2):379–90. https://doi.org/10.1109/TBME.2019.2913752. Epub 2019 Apr 29

Greenhill AEB. A primer of AI in medicine. Tech Gastrointest Endosc. 2020;22:85–9.

Hashimoto DA, Witkowski E, Gao L, Meireles O, Rosman G. Artificial intelligence in Anesthesiology: current techniques, clinical applications, and limitations. Anesthesiology. 2020;132(2):379–94. https://doi.org/10.1097/ALN.0000000000002960.

Hayasaka T, Kawano K, Kurihara K, et al. Creation of an artificial intelligence model for intubation difficulty classification by deep learning (convolutional neural network) using face images: an observational study. J Intensive Care. 2021;9(1):38.

Hemmerling TM. Robots will perform anesthesia in the near future. Anesthesiology. 2020;132(2):219–20.

Ho TK. The random subspace method for constructing decision forests. IEEE Trans Pattern Anal Mach Intell. 1998;20(8):832–44. https://doi.org/10.1109/34.709601.

Hoogenboom SA, Bagci U, Wallace MB. AI in gastroenterology. The current state of play and the potential. How will it affect our practice and when? Tech Innov Gastrointest Endosc. 2020;22:42–7.

Huang S, Cai N, Pacheco PP, Narrandes S, Wang Y, Xu W. Applications of support vector machine (SVM) learning in cancer genomics. Cancer Genomics Proteomics. 2018;15(1):41–51. https://doi.org/10.21873/cgp.20063.

Kaul V, Enslin S, Gross SA. History of artificial intelligence in medicine. Gastrointest Endosc. 2020;92(4):807–12. https://doi.org/10.1016/j.gie.2020.06.040. Epub 2020 Jun 18.

Kharghanian R, Peiravi A, Moradi F. Pain detection from facial images using unsupervised feature learning approach. Annu Int Conf IEEE Eng Med Biol Soc. 2016;2016:419–22.

Kuipers BF, Hart PE, Nilsson NJ. Shakey: from conception to history. AI Mag. 2017;38:88–103.

Kulikowski CA. Beginnings of artificial intelligence in medicine (AIM): computational artifice assisting scientific inquiry and clinical art with reflections on present AIM challenges. Yearb Med Inform. 2019;28:249–56.

Li R, Wu Q, Liu J, et al. Monitoring depth of anesthesia based on hybrid features and recurrent neural network. Front Neurosci, 2020, 14: 26.

Lim H, Kim B, Noh GJ, et al. A deep neural network-based pain classifier using a photoplethysmography signal. Sensors. 2019;19(2):384.

Lin CS, Li YC, Mok MS, Wu CC, Chiu HW, Lin YH. Neural network modeling to predict the hypnotic effect of propofol bolus induction. Proc AMIA Symp. 2002;2002:450–3.

Loeb RG, Cannesson M. Closed-loop anesthesia: ready for prime time? Anesth Analg. 2017;124(2):381–2.

Mintz Y, Brodie R. Introduction to artificial intelligence in medicine. Minim Invasive Ther Allied Technol. 2019;28:73–81.

Moran ME. Evolution of robotic arms. J Robot Surg. 2007;1:103–11.

Murthy VH, Krumholz HM, Gross CP. Participation in cancer clinical trials: race-, sex-, and age-based disparities. JAMA. 2004;291:2720–6.

Ni L, Lu C, Liu N, et al. MANDY: towards a smart primary care chatbot application. In: Chen J, Theeramunkong T, Supnithi T, Tang X, editors. Knowledge and Systems Sciences. KSS Communications in Computer and Information Science, vol. 780. Singapore: Springer; 2017.

Puppe F. Introduction to knowledge systems: mark Stefik. Artif Intell Med. 1997;9:201–3.

Quinlan JR. An empirical comparison of genetic and decision-tree classifiers. In: Machine learning proceedings. Amsterdam: Elsevier; 1988. p. 135–41. https://doi.org/10.1016/b978-0-934613-64-4.50019-0.

Ramesh AN, Kambhampati C, Monson JR, et al. Artificial intelligence in medicine. Ann R Coll Surg Engl. 2004;86:334–8.

Rodriguez P, Cucurull G, Gonalez J, et al. Deep pain: exploiting long short-term memory networks for facial expression classification. IEEE Trans Cybern. 2017;52(5):3314–24.

Sameul AI. Some studies in machine learning using the game of checkers. IBM J Res Dev. 1959;3(3):211–29. https://doi.org/10.1147/rd.33.0210.

Schmidhuber J. Deep learning in neural networks: an overview. Neural Netw. 2015;61:85–117. https://doi.org/10.1016/j.neunet.2014.09.003. Epub 2014 Oct 13.

Shimabukuro DW, Barton CW, Feldman MD, Mataraso SJ, Das R. Effect of a machine learning-based severe sepsis prediction algorithm on patient survival and hospital length of stay: a randomised clinical trial. BMJ Open Respir Res. 2017;4:e000234.

Shortliffe EH, Davis R, Axline SG, et al. Computer-based consultations in clinical therapeutics: explanation and rule acquisition capabilities of the MYCIN system. Comput Biomed Res. 1975;8:303–20.

Su MC. Use of neural networks as medical diagnosis expert systems. Comput Biol Med. 1994;24(6):419–29. https://doi.org/10.1016/0010-4825(94)90040-x.

The Massachusetts General Hospital Laboratory of Computer Science. Using decision support to help explain clinical manifestations of disease. 2023.; http://www.mghlcs.org/projects/dxplain. Accessed 8 Feb 2023.

Urrea C, Mignogna A. Development of an expert system for pre-diagnosis of hypertension, diabetes mellitus type 2 and metabolic syndrome. Health Informatics J. 2020;26(4):2776–91. https://doi.org/10.1177/1460458220937095. Epub 2020 Jul 21.

Vinsard DG, Mori Y, Misawa M, et al. Quality assurance of computer aided detection and diagnosis in colonoscopy. Gastrointest Endosc. 2019;90:55–63.

Weiss S, Kulikowski CA, Safir A. Glaucoma consultation by computer. Comput Biol Med. 1978;8:25–40.

Weizenbaum J. ELIZAda computer program for the study of natural language communication between man and machine. Commun ACM. 1966;9:36–45.

Yang YJ, Bang CS. Application of artificial intelligence in gastroenterology. World J Gastroenterol. 2019;25:1666–83.

Yazhou W, Xicheng C, Dong Y. Advances and perspective of artificial intelligence in clinical area. J Army Med Univ. 2022;44(1):89–102.

Machine Learning and Other Techniques in Artificial Intelligence

Ming Xia

The term "artificial intelligence" (AI) was introduced in the 1950s and was proposed at the beginning as a simple theory of representing human intelligence in machines (Bini 2018). In 1976, Jerrold S. Maxmen predicted that AI would open the "post-doctoral era" in the twenty-first century (Maxmen 1976; Naylor 2018). Today, his prediction has been validated by the rapid development of AI technologies, the exponential growth of mega data sets ("big data"), and the transition of AI from mere theory to practical applications of unprecedented scale (Topol 2019). From AI clothes fitting, to tailor-made health recipes, to voice-controlled smart appliances, to driverless cars, etc., these technologies have greatly improved the human experience in all aspects of clothing, food, housing, and transportation. The combination of AI and anesthesiology has been a trend that cannot be halted. Since AI has been a broad topic embracing various techniques that support its development, it is necessary to introduce machine learning and its algorithms before exploring the existing and probable role of AI in administering high-quality anesthesia.

M. Xia (✉)
Department of Anesthesiology, Shanghai Ninth People's Hospital, Shanghai Jiao Tong University School of Medicine, Shanghai, China
e-mail: xiaming1980@xzhmu.edu.cn

1 Machine Learning, a Key Subfield of AI

Artificial intelligence and machine learning (ML) have been popular topics that draw the attention of people from all walks of life. Nevertheless, the majority oversimplified the relationship between AI and ML. This section illustrates how ML serving as the foundation boosts the development of AI.

Machine learning (ML), as a subset of AI, literally means that machines exhibit empirical "learning" behaviors similar to human intelligence, but at the same time have the ability to learn and improve their own analytical processes through computational algorithms. Those algorithms use large sets of data inputs and outputs to identify behavioral patterns and effectively "learn" them in order to train the machine to make autonomous recommendations or decisions. After constant repetition and modification of the algorithm, the machine becomes able to accept inputs and predict outputs (Bini 2018; Naylor 2018). The output is then compared to a set of known outcomes to evaluate the accuracy of the algorithm, which is then iteratively tuned to refine the ability to predict further outcomes (Haeberle et al. 2019).

Machine learning is closely related to, and often overlaps with, computational statistics, which also focuses on making predictions through the use of computers. Also, machine

M. Xia, H. Jiang (eds.), *Artificial Intelligence in Anesthesiology*,
https://doi.org/10.1007/978-981-99-5925-9_2

learning is closely related to mathematical optimization exercises, which provide the domain of methods, theory, and applications for machine learning. Some people may confuse machine learning with data mining, a subfield that is more focused on exploratory data analysis, or unsupervised learning, which is described below.

While there is a wide variety of machine learning algorithms, data is often more important than the selected algorithm. Various defects may be found in the data collected, including insufficient, poor quality, incorrect, missing, and irrelevant data, and duplicate data values. A dataset is a collection of data values that can be in the form of a CSV file or a spreadsheet. Each column is called a feature and each row is a data point consisting of a specific set of values for each feature. If a dataset holds information about customers, then each row is associated with a specific customer. In the field of data analytics, machine learning is a method for designing complex models and algorithms that play an important role in prediction. Various analytic models help researchers, data scientists, engineers, and analysts to obtain "reliable, repeatable decisions and results" and to discover "hidden insights" by learning from historical relationships and trends in data.

1.1 Types of Machine Learning

As AI techniques continuously upgraded and iterated, the classification of machine learning techniques has also been innovated. By learning problems, machine learning can be classified as supervised learning, unsupervised learning, and reinforcement learning (Russell and Norvig 2009). This type of classification is also commonly used in the study of medicine-related fields. Besides, by hybrid learning problems, it is divided into semi-supervised learning, self-supervised learning, and multi-instance learning (Goodfellow et al. 2016); by statistical inference, it includes inductive learning, deductive inference, and transductive learning; by learning techniques, it can be classified as multi-task learning, active learning, online learning, transfer learning, and ensemble learning. Each of these types of learning algorithms has a range of techniques that can be applied. We will mainly focus on supervised learning, unsupervised learning, and reinforcement learning.

1.1.1 Supervised Learning

Supervised learning is a task-driven process in which the algorithm learns from labeled data, and after understanding the data, it can determine which label should be assigned to the new data by associating patterns with the new unlabeled data. Supervised learning can be divided into two categories: classification and regression. Classification problems are used to predict the category to which the data belongs. Examples of classification in everyday life include spam detection, customer churn prediction, sentiment analysis, and dog breed detection. Examples of regression include house price prediction, stock price prediction, and height-weight prediction. The regression problem predicts values based on previously observed data. When supervised learning is applied in anesthesiology, it can assist to differentiate the patient's anesthesia status, select the best anesthesia, identify potential patients for healthcare, etc. with the help of a decision tree. Normally, supervised learning requires a training dataset and a test dataset. The training dataset allows the machine to analyze and learn the association between the input values and the desired output values, while the test dataset allows to evaluate the performance of the algorithm on new data. In many studies, a large data set is subdivided into a training set and a test set (typically 70% of the data is used for training and 30% for testing) (Hashimoto et al. 2020).

For example, Kendale et al. (2018) underwent a supervised learning study on electronic health record data aiming to identify patients who presented with post-induction hypotension (mean arterial pressure [MAP] below 55 mmHg). The training data set included 70% of the patients and a number of variables such as the American Society of Anesthesiologists (ASA) physical status, age, body mass index (BMI), comorbidities, and medications, and also the patient's blood pressure. The different algorithms used by Kendale et al. (2018) were then able to analyze the training dataset to figure out which variables predict post-induction hypotension. The test dataset was then analyzed to evaluate the accuracy of the algorithm predicting post-induction hypotension in the remaining 30% of patients. Several studies have used external validation such as using separate datasets, to assess the generalizability of the algorithm to other data sources (Wanderer and Rathmell 2018).

1.1.2 Unsupervised Learning

Contrary to supervised learning, unsupervised learning does not label the data but rather is an algorithm that learns or identifies inherent patterns or structures in the dataset. The learned models can be categories, transformations, or probabilities. Such models enable clustering, dimensionality reduction, visualization, probability estimation, and association rule learning on the data. Therefore, it can be useful for exploring new ways to classify patients, drugs, or other groups. Bisgin et al. (2011) used unsupervised learning techniques to mine data from Food and Drug Administration drug labels to identify major themes such as specific adverse events, therapeutic applications, and to automatically classify drugs in order to develop hypotheses for future research. Likewise, unsupervised learning can be helpful in determining the type of drug that is most appropriate for a patient, e.g., an asthma patient who would benefit most from glucocorticoid therapy based on genomic analysis (Hakonarson et al. 2005).

1.1.3 Reinforcement Learning

Reinforcement learning is a machine learning problem in which an intelligent system learns optimal behavioral strategies in continuous interaction with its environment. Examples include driverless cars and automatic delivery systems of anesthetics. The essence of reinforcement learning is to learn the optimal sequential decisions. At each step, the intelligent system observes a state and a reward from the environment and takes action. The environment decides the state and reward for the next moment based on the action taken. The policy to be learned is represented as the action taken in a given state, and the goal is not the maximization of the short-term reward, but the maximization of the long-term cumulative reward. Indeed, today's reinforcement learning problem has become more complex. For example, Padmanabhan et al. (2015) used reinforcement learning to develop an anesthesia controller that collects feedback data from the patient's bispectral index (BIS) and mean arterial pressure (MAP) to control the infusion rate of propofol in a simulated patient model. In this case, achieving BIS and MAP values within a set range gives the algorithm a reward, while values outside this range lead to errors, prompting further optimization of the algorithm.

2 Techniques and Models within Machine Learning

Among the three approaches to machine learning described above, there are various techniques and models. Although a detailed description of the specific methods and algorithms used in machine learning is beyond the scope of this review, it is useful to have an introductory familiarity with the basic concepts of the more general techniques used in artificial intelligence research.

2.1 Fuzzy Logic

The description of fuzzy set theory and fuzzy logic first appeared in 1965 (Zadeh 1965). Although fuzzy logic itself may not necessarily belong to artificial intelligence, it can serve in other frameworks to enhance the application of other functions based on artificial intelligence. Standard logic allows only the concepts of true (value 1.0) and false (value 0.0), but fuzzy logic allows partial truth, for example, values between 0.0 and 1.0. It can be compared to probability theory, where the probability of a statement being true ("A pancreaticoduodenectomy will be scheduled tomorrow") is evaluated against the degree to which a statement is true ("The probability of scheduling a pancreaticoduodenectomy tomorrow is 80%"). The purpose of this technique is to simulate the human decision-making process for ambiguous or imprecise information (Hashimoto et al. 2020).

Fuzzy logic relies on rule-based systems such as the "if… then" systems which are commonly adopted in control systems because precise mathematical functions do not accurately model phenomena. For instance, an anesthesia monitor for detecting hypovolemia was developed on the foundation of fuzzy logic to approximate the appearance of mild, moderate, and severe hypovolemia according to normalized values of heart rate (HR), blood pressure, and pulse volume which were classified as mild, moderate, and severe. The monitor employs rules established on fuzzy logic, for example, "If (electrocardiogram-HR is mild) and (blood pressure is mild) and (pulse volume is severe), then (hypovolemia is moderate)" (Baig et al. 2011).

The development of such rules requires the input of human experts to determine an appropriate set of rules that can be followed by machines. Early research on fuzzy logic and other adaptive control mechanisms laid the groundwork for exploring more modern approaches to imprecise information or incomplete data. AI methods have been introduced in recent research in this field to facilitate the evaluation and use of data to trigger the rule functions of fuzzy systems. Therefore, while research in fuzzy logic systems remains ongoing, particularly in control systems for applications such as drug delivery, advances in AI research have targeted the use of more data-driven techniques in machine learning to enable the goals first explored by researchers in fuzzy logic.

2.2 Classical Machine Learning

The task performance of machine learning relied on features or attributes of the data. Similar to that in statistical analysis, features could be regarded as the independent variables in a logistic regression. In classical machine learning, features are chosen by experts to guide the algorithms in analyzing complex data.

Decision tree learning is a supervised learning algorithm that can be used to perform either classification (classification trees) or regression tasks (regression trees). As is implied by its name, this set of techniques uses flowchart-like tree models with multiple branch points to identify a target value or classification of an input. Each node within a tree has a specified value, with the final node representing the endpoint and the cumulative probability of reaching this endpoint based on the previous decisions. Hu et al. used decision trees to predict the total consumption of patient-controlled analgesia (PCA) consumption by characteristics such as patient demographics, vital signs, medical history, surgery type, and PCA doses consumed, and finally, in turn, using such techniques to optimize PCA dosing regimens (Hu et al. 2012).

The k-nearest neighbor algorithms are a set of supervised learning algorithms that evaluate training data geometrically and then identify whether additional input data belongs to a certain category in light of the closest training examples plotted closest to it (according to Euclidian distance). Depending on the specific approach used, this may be based on a single nearest point (1-nearest neighbor) or on the weights of a set of points (k-nearest neighbor). Support vector machines are another type of supervised learning algorithm that plays a useful role in classification and regression. They map training data in space and optimize the classification of the data by hyperplanes into representative groups or clusters. Subsequently, new data are divided according to their location in the space relative to the hyperplane (Hastie et al. 2016).

2.3 Neural Networks and Deep Learning

Deep learning, known as deep structured learning, hierarchical learning, or deep machine learning as well, explores artificial neural networks and related machine learning algorithms encompassing more than one hidden layer.

Using neural networks to accomplish tasks of machine learning has been quite popular in these days. The inspiration for neural networks originates from biological nervous systems that process signals in layers of computational units (neurons). Each network is composed of an input layer of neurons that consists of features representing the data. Among all layers of neurons, at least one hidden layer performs different mathematical transformations of the input features, and an output layer produces the result. There are multiple connections between neurons lying between each layer. Those neurons are parameterized with different weights based on the input–output maps. Therefore, neural networks are a framework within which different machine learning algorithms can perform to accomplish a specific task, for example, image recognition and data classification.

Modern neural network architectures have been extended to allow deep learning, that is, the use of many layers of neural networks to learn more complex patterns than can be discerned by simple one- or two-layer networks. Some of the most successful deep learning methods are concerned with artificial neural networks that are inspired by the biological models proposed by Nobel laureates David H. Hubel and Torsten Wiesel in 1959, who identified two types of cells in the primary visual cortex: simple and complex cells. Various artificial neural networks can be regarded as cascade models of cell types motivated by these biological observations (Weng et al. 1992).

Fukushima's Neocognitron introduced convolutional neural networks that were trained in part by unsupervised learning with human-guided features on the neural plane. LeCun et al. (1989) applied supervised backpropagation to such architectures. Weng et al. (1992) published the convolutional neural network Cresceptron for identifying 3D objects from images of cluttered scenes and for segmenting such objects from images (LeCun et al. 1989; Weng et al. 1993).

Igor Aizenberg and colleagues in 2000 proposed the use of the expression "deep learning" in the context of artificial neural networks. A Google Ngram chart shows that the use of the term has become popular since 2000. More attention was drawn to a 2006 paper by Geoffrey Hinton and Ruslan Salakhutdinov, who showed how multilayer feedforward neural networks can be effectively pre-trained layer by layer, treating each layer in turn as an unsupervised restricted Boltzmann machine, and then fine-tuned using supervised backpropagation. Schmidhuber had already implemented a very similar idea for the more general case of unsupervised deep recurrent neural networks in 1992, and also experimentally demonstrated its benefits in terms of accelerating supervised learning (Aizenberg et al. 2000; Schmidhuber 2015; Hinton 2007).

The subtypes of deep learning networks one might encounter are convolutional neural networks as well as recurrent neural networks. Convolutional neural networks can process data consisting of multiple arrays, and recurrent neural networks are designed to analyze sequential data such as speech. Generally, features in classical machine learning are handcrafted. Whereas, deep learning self-learns features are based on the data itself. Specifically, deep learning analyzes all available features in the training set to determine which features can best perform a specific task for a deep neural network such as identifying objects from images. Therefore, deep learning may be a powerful tool that can be used to analyze very large datasets where handcrafted features are not sufficient and/or do not yield effective results. One of the promises of deep learning is to replace handcrafted features with efficient algorithms for unsupervised or semi-supervised feature learning and hierarchical feature extraction.

Considering their flexibility in analyzing different types of data, neural networks are now being applied to other subfields of artificial intelligence, including natural language processing and computer vision. Presently, neural networks have also been combined with anesthesia, for example, depth of anesthesia monitoring and control of anesthesia delivery.

2.4 Bayesian Methods

Baye's theorem describes the probability of an event based on previous knowledge or data about factors that may affect that event. In many studies in the medical literature, a frequentist approach to statistics is applied, among which hypothesis testing is based on the frequency of events occurring in a given sample of data as a representation of the study population of interest. However, a Bayesian method uses the known previous probability distributions of events, as well as probability distributions stood for in a given data set (Bidhendi Yarandi et al. 2020).

Many techniques in artificial intelligence are based on Bayes' theorem, due to the fact that the theorem allows modeling of uncertainty and iterative updating or learning as new data becomes available. Bayesian techniques are currently used in many common tasks, such as spam filtering, financial modeling, and evaluation of clinical tests. Although it is beyond the scope of this review to delve into specific Bayesian methods, Bayesian methods like Bayesian networks, Hidden Markov Models, and Kalman filters are being used with increasing frequency in the medical literature (van den Berg et al. 2017; Kukacka 2010).

3 Conclusion

Artificial intelligence, machine learning, and deep learning, at their root, are all related to machine perception, the ability to interpret sensory data. The two main ways we interpret things are by naming our senses; for example, we hear a sound and say "that is my daughter's voice"; or we see a cloud of photons and say "that is my mother's face." Even if things remain unknown to us, we can still recognize their similarities and dissimilarities to the things we perceive. For example, when you see two faces, you know they are mother and daughter even without knowing their names, or you hear two voices and know they are from the same city or state by their accents. The algorithm trains names of things by supervised learning and clustering of things by unsupervised learning. The difference between supervised and unsupervised learning is whether you work with a labeled training set or not. The labels you add to the data are the results you are concerned about, for example, you try to identify people in images or identify spam, which are unstructured text. Maybe you are reviewing time series data, which is a string of numbers, but what you intend to acquire is whether the next instance in the time series will be higher or lower.

Thus, deep learning works with other algorithms that can help with classification, clustering, and prediction. Such ability is trained by learning to automatically read the signal or structure in the data. When deep learning algorithms are trained, they make a prediction based on the data, measure their prediction errors against the training set, and then correct their predictions in a way that enhances their prediction accuracy. This process is optimization.

After all, with deep learning, it is possible to classify, cluster, or predict any data that one has, including images, video, sound, text and DNA, and time series. In other words, anything that humans can perceive and that technology can digitize can be processed as described above. In this way, the ability of humans to analyze what is happening in the world has doubled several times. With deep learning, humans essentially give society the ability to behave more intelligently, and to explain exactly what is happening in the world around them through software, and this ability will continue to improve as technology evolves.

References

Aizenberg I, Aizenberg NN, Vandewalle JPL. Multi-valued and universal binary neurons: theory, learning and applications. Springer Science & Business Media; 2000.

Baig MM, Gholamhosseini H, Kouzani A, Harrison MJ. Anaesthesia monitoring using fuzzy logic. J Clin Monit Comput. 2011;25:339–47.

Bidhendi Yarandi R, Mohammad K, Zeraati H, Ramezani Tehrani F, Mansournia MA. Bayesian methods for clinicians. Med J Islam Repub Iran. 2020;13(34):78. https://doi.org/10.34171/mjiri.34.78.

Bini SA. Artificial intelligence, machine learning, deep learning, and cognitive computing: what do these terms mean and how will they impact health care? J Arthroplast. 2018;33(8):2358–61. https://doi.org/10.1016/j.arth.2018.02.067.

Bisgin H, Liu Z, Fang H, Xu X, Tong W. Mining FDA drug labels using an unsupervised learning technique–topic modeling. BMC Bioinformatics. 2011;12(Suppl 10):S11.

Goodfellow I, Bengio Y, Courville A. Deep learning. Cambridge: The MIT Press; 2016.

Haeberle HS, Helm JM, Navarro SM, et al. Artificial intelligence and machine learning in lower extremity arthroplasty: a review. J Arthroplast. 2019;34(10):2201–3. https://doi.org/10.1016/j.arth.2019.05.055.

Hakonarson H, Bjornsdottir US, Halapi E, Bradfield J, Zink F, Mouy M, Helgadottir H, Gudmundsdottir AS, Andrason H, Adalsteinsdottir AE, Kristjansson K, Birkisson I, Arnason T, Andresdottir M, Gislason D, Gislason T, Gulcher JR, Stefansson K. Profiling of genes expressed in peripheral blood mononuclear cells predicts glucocorticoid sensitivity in asthma patients. Proc Natl Acad Sci U S A. 2005;102:14789–94.

Hashimoto DA, Witkowski E, Gao L, Meireles O, Rosman G. Artificial intelligence in Anesthesiology: current techniques, clinical applications, and limitations. Anesthesiology. 2020;132(2):379–94. https://doi.org/10.1097/ALN.0000000000002960.

Hastie T, Tibshirani R, Friedman J. Support vector machines and flexible discriminants, the elements of statistical learning: data mining, inference, and prediction. New York: Springer; 2016. p. 417–58.

Hinton GE. Learning multiple layers of representation. Trends Cogn Sci. 2007;11:428–34.

Hu YJ, Ku TH, Jan RH, Wang K, Tseng YC, Yang SF. Decision tree-based learning to predict patient controlled analgesia consumption and readjustment. BMC Med Inform Decis Mak. 2012;12:131.

Kendale S, Kulkarni P, Rosenberg AD, Wang J. Supervised machine-learning predictive analytics for prediction of postinduction hypotension. Anesthesiology. 2018;129:675–88.

Kukacka M. Bayesian methods in artificial intelligence, WDS'10 proceedings of contributed papers; 2010. p. 25–30.

LeCun Y, Boser B, Denker JS, Henderson D, Howard RE, Hubbard W, Jackel LD. Backpropagation applied to handwritten zip code recognition. Neural Comput. 1989;1(4):541–51.

Maxmen JS. The post-physician era: medicine in the twenty-first century. Hoboken: Wiley; 1976.

Naylor CD. On the prospects for a (deep) learning health care system. JAMA. 2018;320(11):1099–100. https://doi.org/10.1001/jama.2018.11103.

Padmanabhan R, Meskin N, Haddad WM. Closed-loop control of anesthesia and mean arterial pressure using reinforcement learning. Biomed Signal Process Control. 2015;22:54–64.

Russell S, Norvig P. Artificial intelligence: a modern approach. 3rd ed. Upper Saddle River: Prentice Hall; 2009.

Jürgen Schmidhuber (2015) Google Ngram chart of the usage of the expression "deep learning".https://plus.google.com/100849856540000067209/posts/7N6z251w2Wd?pid=6127540521703625346&oid=100849856540000067209.

Topol EJ. High-performance medicine: the convergence of human and artificial intelligence. Nat Med. 2019;25:44–56. https://doi.org/10.1038/s41591-018-0300-7.

van den Berg JP, Eleveld DJ, De Smet T, van den Heerik AVM, van Amsterdam K, Lichtenbelt BJ, Scheeren TWL, Absalom AR, Struys MMRF. Influence of Bayesian optimization on the performance of propofol target-controlled infusion. Br J Anaesth. 2017;119:918–27.

Wanderer JP, Rathmell JP. Machine learning for anesthesiologists: a primer. Anesthesiology. 2018;129:A29.

Weng J, Ahuja N, Huang TS. Cresceptron: a self-organizing neural network which grows adaptively. In: Proc. international joint conference on neural networks, Baltimore, Maryland, vol. I; 1992. p. 576–81.

Weng J, Ahuja N, Huang TS. Learning recognition and segmentation of 3-D objects from 2-D images. In: Proc. 4th international conf. computer vision. Berlin: IEEE; 1993. p. 121–8.

Zadeh LA. Fuzzy sets. Inf Control. 1965;8:338–53.

Assistance of Artificial Intelligence in Ultrasound-Based Procedures

Chenyu Jin

The urgent requirement for the use and development of ultrasound (US) techniques has been realized for a long time. Compared with computed tomography (CT) and magnetic resonance imaging (MRI), US has the advantages of being non-invasive, less costly, and having no radiation exposure. Therefore, it is commonly used for screening and diagnosis (Reddy et al. 2008). Except for the common use in point-of-care testing in emergency medical treatment and palliative care, it is now combined with laboratory tests, serving as the multi-biomarker strategy for predicting the clinical outcome.

However, image quality control remains to be a critical defect of US image acquisition. For one thing, the image acquisition of CT and MRI is performed automatically with a specific patient, a fixed measurement time, and consistent image settings. Whereas, US imaging is acquired through manual sweep scanning, indicating that the image quality depends on the skill levels of the examiners. Moreover, the image quality and diagnostic accuracy may be affected by acoustic shadows caused by obstructions including bones (Feldman et al. 2009).

Artificial intelligence (AI), including machine learning and deep learning, has developed rapidly in recent years and is increasingly being incorporated into medical research and applications (Asada et al. 2021). Deep learning is a leading subset of machine learning, defined as the use of convolutional neural networks (CNNs) to learn non-programmatically from large amounts of data (LeCun et al. 2015). This state-of-the-art technique offers the potential to perform tasks more rapidly and accurately than humans in specific areas such as imaging and pattern recognition (Chen et al. 2021; Esteva et al. 2017). In particular, medical imaging analysis is compatible with AI, where classification, detection, and segmentation are used as the fundamental tasks in AI-based imaging analyses. In addition, many AI-driven medical devices have been approved by the US Food and Drug Administration (FDA) for clinical use (Wu et al. 2021).

More than a dozen papers describe the use of artificial intelligence techniques to assist in performing ultrasound-based procedures, and neural networks are the most common method to achieve ultrasound image classification. Smistad et al. used inguinal ultrasound images from 15 patients to train convolutional neural networks to identify the femoral artery or vein while distinguishing it from other similar ultrasound images that may appear such as muscle, bone, or even acoustic shadow. Further investigation of this network revealed that it prioritized the analysis of horizontal edges in ultrasound over vertical edges to identify blood vessels with an average accuracy of 94.5% ± 2.9% (Smistad et al. 2016).

C. Jin (✉)
Department of Anesthesiology, Shanghai Ninth People's Hospital, Shanghai Jiao Tong University School of Medicine, Shanghai, China

M. Xia, H. Jiang (eds.), *Artificial Intelligence in Anesthesiology*,
https://doi.org/10.1007/978-981-99-5925-9_3

Apart from structure-specific detection in ultrasound images, researchers have used neural networks to assist in identifying vertebral levels and other anatomical landmarks for epidural placement. Pesteie et al. (2018) used convolutional neural networks to automatically identify the anterior base of the vertebral lamina, while Hetherington et al. (2017) used convolutional neural networks to automatically identify the sacrum and L1–L5 vertebrae and vertebral spaces from ultrasound images in real time with an accuracy up to 95%.

1 US Image Preprocessing

Ultrasound imaging usually exhibits low spatial resolution and many artifacts due to ultrasound diffraction. These features affect not only the examination and diagnosis of ultrasound, but also artificial intelligence-based image processing and recognition. Therefore, several ultrasound image preprocessing methods have been proposed that eliminate the noise that hinders accurate feature extraction prior to ultrasound image processing. Two methods for ultrasound image quality improvement and acoustic shadow detection will be presented here.

First, several techniques have been developed that can improve ultrasound image quality by reducing speckles, clutter, and other artifacts. Ultrasonic beam steering using an array of transducers has been proposed to acquire real-time spatial composite imaging of multiple multi-angle scans of an object. In addition, harmonic imaging using endogenously generated low frequencies has been proposed to reduce attenuation and improve image contrast. Ultrasound image enhancement using conventional image processing methods has been reported. Despeckling is a representative research topic for filtering or removing point-like artifacts in ultrasound imaging. With this approach, the causes of image quality degradation are eliminated at the root cause during the ultrasound image generation stage or noise features are modeled after careful inspection during ultrasound image generation. Current approaches to improving ultrasound image quality using machine learning or deep learning include improving despeckle performance, as well as improving overall image quality. One significant advantage of this data-driven approach is that there is no need to create a model for each domain. However, improving ultrasound image quality requires a large amount of targeted, high-quality training data, which can present critical problems in clinical applications due to the general difficulty of preparing such a dataset.

Several techniques have been developed that can improve ultrasound image quality by reducing speckles, clutter, and other artifacts during image acquisition. Ultrasonic beam steering using an array of transducers has been proposed to acquire real-time spatial composite imaging of multi-angle scans of an object. In addition, harmonic imaging using endogenously generated low frequencies has been proposed to reduce attenuation and improve image contrast. Ultrasound image enhancement using conventional image processing methods has been reported. Despeckling is a representative research topic for filtering or removing point-like artifacts in ultrasound imaging. With this approach, during the ultrasound image generation stage, the causes of image quality degradation are eliminated at the root cause or noise features are modeled after careful inspection. Current approaches to improving ultrasound image quality using machine learning or deep learning include the improvement of despeckle performance and overall image quality. One significant advantage of this data-driven approach is that there is no need to create a model for each domain. However, improving ultrasound image quality requires a large amount of targeted, high-quality training data, which is difficult to prepare, and therefore, critical problems in clinical applications may sprout.

Acoustic shadow detection is also a well-known method for ultrasound image preprocessing. Acoustic shadow is one of the most representative artifacts, caused by several reflectors blocking the ultrasound beam propagating in a straight line from the transducer. Some useful artifacts, such as the comet tail artifact (B-line), can provide clues to help diagnose COVID-19 infection in point-of-care lung ultrasound. However, its presentation as black in this region is similar to missing information, which hinders the presentation of examination results and AI-based image recognition of the target organ in US imaging. Therefore, acoustic shadow detection prior to US imaging analysis can help determine whether the acquired images are suitable as input data. Conventional image processing methods for detecting acoustic shadows include automatic geometric and statistical methods (break detection using brightness values along the scan line), and random walk-based methods. In these methods, parameters and models need to be carefully changed to cope with shifts in the domain. However, deep learning-based methods can be applied to a much wider range of domains. The preparation of training datasets remains challenging due to the high cost and difficulty of pixel-level annotation of acoustic shadows due to their translucent nature and blurred boundaries.

2 Algorithms for US Imaging Analysis

The specialized algorithms for US imaging analysis to overwhelm the noisy artifacts and the instability of the viewpoint and cross-section owing to manual operation will be introduced in this section.

Classification, detection, and segmentation are commonly used as basic algorithms for US imaging analysis. Classification evaluates one or more labels across the image and is often used as a standard scan plane for screening or diagnosis in US imaging analysis. ResNet and Visual Geometry Group (VGG) are examples of classification methods. Detection primarily serves to evaluate lesions and anatomical structures. YOLO and the single-shot multibox detector (SSD) are popular detection algorithms. Segmentation is used for further accurate pixel measurements of lesions and organ structures, as well as exponential calculations of length, area, and volume. U-Net and DeepLab are representative algorithms for segmentation. These standard algorithms are often used as baselines to evaluate the performance of specialized algorithms for US imaging analysis.

There are specialized algorithms for US imaging analysis to address performance degradation due to noise artifacts. Cropping-segmentation-calibration (CSC) and multi-frame + cylinder method (MFCY) use time series information to reduce noise artifacts and perform accurate segmentation in US videos. Deep attention networks have also been proposed to improve segmentation performance in US imaging, such as attention-guided dual path networks and a U-Net-based network that combines a channel attention module and VGG. A framework based on contrast learning and a framework based on generative adversarial networks (GAN) for progressive learning has been reported to improve boundary prediction in US imaging.

Critical problems caused by the instability of views and cross-sections often become apparent when calculating clinical metrics with segmentation methods. One traditional ultrasound image processing method is the reconstruction of three-dimensional (3D) volumes. Traditional direct segmentation methods of 3D volumes, including 3D U-Net, are useful for accurate volume quantification; however, labeling them is very expensive and time-consuming. Interactive few-shot Stiamese networks use Stiamese networks and recurrent neural networks to train 3D segmentation from a few annotated two-dimensional (2D) ultrasound images. Another research topic is the extraction of 2D US images involving standard scanning planes from 3D ultrasound volume. The iterative transformation network aims to guide the current plane toward the position of the standard scanning planes in the 3D ultrasound volume. In addition, Duque et al. proposed a semi-automatic segmentation algorithm for free-hand 3D ultrasound volume, which is a continuous 2D cross-section formed by using an encoder-decoder architecture with 2D ultrasound images and several 2D labels (Gonzalez Duque et al. 2020).

3 Clinical Application of US Images Using AI Techniques

3.1 Vessel Detection in US Images

Vessel segmentation in ultrasound images can be applied to aid in deep vein thrombosis detection, anesthesia guidance, and catheter placement. The goal of vessel detection in this work is to determine the location and size of the vessels in the image. Some segmentation and tracking methods require this as an initialization. In reference (Smistad and Lindseth 2016), a real-time vascular detection method was introduced that eliminates the need for manual initialization. This method uses a graphics processing unit (GPU) to perform ellipse fitting on each pixel of the image. However, this method is biased in differentiating between vessels and non-vessels when changing user settings, such as on ultrasound scanners and in people with more subcutaneous fat tissue because of the increased number of reverberation artifacts. In addition, this method is only used to detect a single vessel per image.

Smistad and Lindseth (2016) proposed to use a similar ellipse fitting method to find vessel candidate regions and pass it to a deep neural network classifier to determine if the region contains a vessel (Fig. 1). This detection method provides the location and size, and can also be used as a vessel segmentation method, assuming the vessel is elliptical. The method is also capable of detecting multiple blood vessels simultaneously.

3.1.1 Vessel Model

Each vessel is modelled as an ellipse with center $c = [cx, cy]$ and major and minor radius a and b. The point pi and its normal ni of point i on an ellipse of N equally distributed points can be calculated with the following equations:

$$\alpha_i = \frac{2\pi i}{\mathrm{N}} \tag{1}$$

$$\mathrm{d}_i = \left[\mathrm{a}\cos(\alpha_i), \mathrm{b}\sin(\alpha_i)\right] \tag{2}$$

$$\mathrm{p}_i = \mathrm{c} + \mathrm{d}_i \tag{3}$$

$$\mathrm{n}_i = \frac{\left[\mathrm{b}\cos(\alpha_i), \mathrm{a}\sin(\alpha_i)\right]}{\left\|\left[\mathrm{b}\cos(\alpha_i), \mathrm{a}\sin(\alpha_i)\right]\right\|} \tag{4}$$

3.1.2 Vessel Candidate Search

At first, using convolution with a Gaussian mask ($\sigma = 0.5$ mm) blur the image and then the image gradients G are calculated using a central difference scheme. For given radii a and b, the vessel score S is calculated as the average dot product of the outward normal ni and the corresponding image gradient at N points on the ellipse. The equation is shown below:

$$\mathrm{S}(\mathrm{c,a,b}) = \frac{1}{N}\sum_{i=0}^{N-1} n_i nG(p_i) \tag{5}$$

For each pixel, different major radii a from 3.5 mm to 6 mm, flattening factors f from 0 to 0.5 (minor radius $b = (1-f)$ a) and $N = 32$ samples of ellipses were used to calculate the vascular score. The increment of radius was 0.25 mm and the flattening factor was 0.1. The highest-scoring ellipse was selected for each pixel. The best score and values a and b for each pixel were stored. Any candidate vessel with a score lower than 1.5 was discarded, which was a low threshold so that vessels with low contrast would not be discarded,

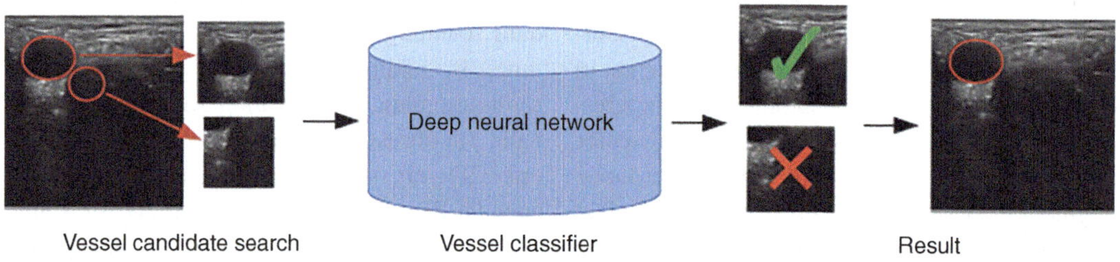

Fig. 1 The ellipse fitting method proposed by Smistad et al., where vessel candidate regions are found and passed to a deep neural network classifier to determine if the region contains a vessel

but several nonvascular regions would be included. Then, candidate vessels are sorted according to their scores from highest to lowest. These vessels are then processed in order and if the center is not within another already accepted vessel candidate structure, this vessel candidate structure is accepted. Any candidate vessel that overlaps with a previously accepted candidate vessel is discarded.

3.1.3 Vessel Classifier

The next step is to run each blood vessel candidate image through a deep convolutional neural network classifier to identify whether the image belongs to a blood vessel or not. Caffe was used as the underlying framework for classifier training and testing, and at the same time, the vessel candidate search was implemented by the FAST medical image computing framework (Jia et al. 2014; Smistad et al. 2015).

The AlexNet network was initially used and progressively simplified by removing convolution-pooling blocks and reducing the number of convolutions, while keeping the accuracy of the verification. The network was simplified mainly to increase the speed at which the test could run, which was important to achieve real-time performance. The final vessel classification network consists of two convolutional layers, one normalization layer, two max pooling layers, and three fully connected layers. In addition, rectified linear units (ReLU), which have been shown to improve training, were used as nonlinear activation units for the convolutional and fully connected (FC) layers. Therefore, the network consists of a total of 13 layers, including the ReLU layer. In addition, the network is trained using the softmax loss layer. The size of the data layer was fixed to 110 × 110 pixels. During the training process, random patches of size 110 × 110 were cropped from the 128 × 128 vascular candidate images to prevent overfitting. This technique improved the accuracy by 1%. The average image was computed from the training data and subtracted from the input image. The first convolution layer had 9 convolutions of size 11 × 11 pixels and the second convolutional layer had 32 convolutions of size 15 × 15. The maximum set was done on a 3 × 3 patch. Local response normalization (LRN) was used after the first convolution layer with the same parameters as in the research of Krizhevsky et al. Dropout was used on the fully connected layer with a probability of 0.5. The network was trained using stochastic gradient descent with a batch size of 128, momentum of 0.9, and weight decay of 0.0005. The base learning rate was 0.01 with a sigmoid learning rate decay.

3.1.4 Outcomes

The convolutions learned by the neural network show that the first convolutional layer learns to detect horizontal edges and the second layer learns to recognize horizontal edges with different patterns. It seems that the trained neural network did not find the vertical edges in the ultrasound images important. This seems reasonable considering that vertical edges tend to be weaker or disappear in ultrasound images.

The leave-one-subject-out method of cross-validation was used, so 14 subjects were used for training and 1 subject was reserved for validation. The average classification accuracy for cross-validation was 94.5% with a standard deviation of 2.9. This was calculated using a discrimination threshold of 0.5 for the softmax output of the vessel classifier (Smistad et al. 2016).

3.2 Automatic Localization of the Needle Target for Ultrasound-Guided Epidural Injections

Epidural anesthesia is a common method used in obstetrics and chronic pain management. Epidural anesthesia involves placing a local anesthetic needle into the epidural space between the ligamentum flavum and the dura mater, with the patient in a sitting or lying position with an arched back to extend the intervertebral gap. Studies have shown that the two positions are indistinguishable in terms of efficacy, operative time, and patient comfort level. Conventional epidural anesthesia is guided by palpation and loss-of-resistance technique or is performed under fluoroscopy. The traditional loss-of-resistance has a failure rate of 6–20% (Kim et al. 2012). Failure is defined as poor or no postoperative pain relief, usually due to needle misplacement. In some cases, the needle tip overshoots as it passes through the epidural space, piercing the dura, which can lead to headaches and other complications. In addition, fluoroscopy has significant shortcomings, such as exposing the patient to ionizing radiation, and therefore the use of fluoroscopy for epidural anesthesia is contraindicated during labor and delivery.

Fortunately, US technology has recently been used to facilitate spinal needle injections and lumbar epidural anesthesia, and the clinical feasibility of using US-guided injections has been investigated (Conroy et al. 2013). Generally, US images are often difficult to interpret due to the complexity of anatomical structures compared to other imaging techniques, and images are often affected by speckle noise, acoustic clutter, reverberation artifacts, and shadowing. Although beam formation and image filtering algorithms are continuously improved in order to promote the overall image quality, image interpretation remains a key challenge with a steep learning curve for novices. Moreover, current US-guided injection systems provide limited guidance to physicians, such as accurate positioning of the needle target prior to needle insertion and guidance of the needle during the procedure. Therefore, a system to automatically identify and locate needle targets in spinal US images is needed. Such a guidance system has potential benefits to patients, such as increased analgesic use and effectiveness and reduced incidence and severity of associated complications. In particular, the goal of the guidance system is to allow any operator, including novice ultrasound users to correctly identify the location of injections in different patients. Studies have shown that ultrasound guidance can reduce the learning time of novices, as well as the number of needle insertions required before reaching the target. The expected benefit of studies is to reduce complications and perform successful anesthesia in most patients by improving the accuracy of needle positioning and operator confidence and success rates.

In the study, Pesteie et al. illustrate their goal of developing a machine learning technique that would help the operator to accurately locate the needle target in US images before or during needle insertion (Pesteie et al. 2018). They propose a convolutional network architecture identifying and localizing the epidural space in paramedian US images of the lumbar spine (Pesteie et al. 2018). They introduce a feature intensification technique that combines the convolutional feature maps obtained from convolutional layers with multiscale local directional Hadamard features. Since the multiscale Hadamard features are sensitive to the directionality of US echoes from the vertebral surface in the US image, the enhancement provides the deep network with a unique set of directional features from the sequence domain in addition to the feature maps automatically obtained from the spatial domain. In addition, they demonstrate that the enhanced Hadamard features are not automatically learned by deep networks with the same number of convolutional layers and kernels. Therefore, the enhanced features are not redundant. The impact of feature enhancement on pixel-level classification performance is shown by evaluating the accuracy of the proposed network against a conventional CNN architecture with the same number of convolutional layers and kernels. Furthermore, they display that augmenting Hadamard features with convolutional feature maps improves the accuracy of target localization compared to the localization results of template matching and state-of-the-art deep networks for biomedical image segmentation.

Bowness et al. demonstrate the clinical utility of an assistive AI system in aiding the identification of anatomical structures on ultrasound during ultrasound-guided regional anesthesia (Bowness et al. 2021). The system they assessed is *ScanNav Anatomy Peripheral Nerve Block* (Intelligent Ultrasound Ltd), facilitating the identification of anatomical structures on ultrasound for the purpose of ultrasound-guided regional anesthesia (UGRA). The evaluation was conducted from a clinical perspective, with experts in the field rating the overall performance of the system, and the assessment focused on whether the system is helpful in identifying relevant anatomical structures and whether it helps less experienced physicians to confirm the correct ultrasound view. Although it must be validated by further studies, the results show promise for the accuracy and clinical utility of the system—especially for non-experts in UGRA, as AI technology can aid the learning and practice of clinicians who regularly practice clinical anatomy but need further anatomical knowledge or skills in ultrasonic anatomical interpretation (Bowness et al. 2021).

References

Asada K, Kaneko S, Takasawa K, Machino H, Takahashi S, Shinkai N, Shimoyama R, Komatsu M, Hamamoto R. Integrated analysis of whole genome and epigenome data using machine learning technology: toward the establishment of precision oncology. Front Oncol. 2021;11:666937.

Bowness J, Varsou O, Turbitt L, Burkett-St LD. Identifying anatomical structures on ultrasound: assistive artificial intelligence in ultrasound-guided regional anesthesia. Clin Anat. 2021;34(5):802–9. https://doi.org/10.1002/ca.23742. Epub 2021 May 11.

Chen Y, Avitabile P, Page C, Dodson J. A polynomial based dynamic expansion and data consistency assessment and modification for cylindrical shell structures. Mech Syst Signal Process. 2021;154:107574.

Conroy P, Luyet C, McCartney C, McHardy P. Real-time ultrasound-guided spinal anaesthesia: a prospective observational study of a new approach. Anesthesiol Res Pract. 2013;2013:1–7.

Esteva A, Kuprel B, Novoa RA, Ko J, Swetter SM, Blau HM, Thrun S. Dermatologist-level classification of skin cancer with deep neural networks. Nature. 2017;542:115–8.

Feldman MK, Katyal S, Blackwood MS. US artifacts. Radiographics. 2009;29:1179–89.

Gonzalez Duque V, Al Chanti D, Crouzier M, Nordez A, Lacourpaille L, Mateus D. Spatio-temporal consistency and negative label transfer for 3D freehand US segmentation. In: Proceedings of the international conference on medical image computing and computer-assisted intervention, Lima, Peru, vol. 4–8; 2020. p. 710–20.

Hetherington J, Lessoway V, Gunka V, Abolmaesumi P, Rohling R. SLIDE: automatic spine level identification system using a deep convolutional neural network. Int J Comput Assist Radiol Surg. 2017;12:1189–98.

Jia Y, Shelhamer E, Donahue J, Karayev S, Long J, Girshick R, Guadarrama S, Darrell T. Caffe: convolutional architecture for fast feature embedding. In: Proceedings of the ACM international conference on multimedia; 2014. p. 675–8.

Kim SW, Kim YM, Kim SH, Chung MH, Choi YR, Choi EM. Comparison of loss of resistance technique between Epidrum® and conventional method for identifying the epidural space. Korean J Anesthesiol. 2012;62(4):322–6. https://doi.org/10.4097/kjae.2012.62.4.322. Epub 2012 Apr 23.

LeCun Y, Bengio Y, Hinton G. Deep learning. Nature. 2015;521:436–44.

Pesteie M, Lessoway V, Abolmaesumi P, Rohling RN. Automatic localization of the needle target for ultrasound-guided epidural injections. IEEE Trans Med Imaging. 2018;37:81–92.

Reddy UM, Filly RA, Copel JA. Prenatal imaging: ultrasonography and magnetic resonance imaging. Obstet Gynecol. 2008;112:145–57.

Smistad E, Lindseth F. Real-time automatic artery segmentation, reconstruction and registration for ultrasound-guided regional anaesthesia of the femoral nerve. IEEE Trans Med Imaging. 2016;35(3):752–61.

Smistad E, Bozorgi M, Lindseth F. FAST: framework for heterogeneous medical image computing and visualization. Int J Comput Assist Radiol Surg. 2015;10(11):1811–22.

Smistad E, Lovstakken L, Carneiro G, Mateus D, Peter L, Bradley A, Tavares J, Belagiannis V, Papa JP, Nascimento JC, Loog M, Lu Z, Cardoso JS, Cornebise J. Vessel detection in ultrasound images using deep convolutional neural networks, med image comput comput assist inter. Springer; 2016. p. 30–8.

Wu E, Wu K, Daneshjou R, Ouyang D, Ho DE, Zou J. How medical AI devices are evaluated: limitations and recommendations from an analysis of FDA approvals. Nat Med. 2021;27:582–4.

Artificial Intelligence in Anesthesia Control and Monitoring

Bei Pei

Artificial intelligence (AI) is increasingly being used in clinical anesthesia, and researchers are using algorithms to dig information from patients' perioperative data, process and analyze them from multi-dimensions, after which predictive models are built to dynamically predict perioperative adverse events.

The depth of anesthesia (DOA) is associated with morbidity, mortality, postoperative adverse events, and related organ damage. Therefore, maintaining the appropriate DOA in the perioperative period is of great significance for clinical anesthesia. Currently, the monitoring of perioperative anesthetic depth uses BIS. Maintaining BIS at 40–60 can avoid intraoperative awareness and deep anesthesia, but the monitoring may be influenced because there is a time lag and BIS may be easily interfered by the electrotome. There are researches exploring the monitoring of the DOA according to the patient's original electroencephalography (EEG). Due to the complex changes of EEG under different anesthesia states, it is difficult to effectively assess the DOA by extracting a single feature, while multiple effective features can be extracted from EEG with the help of AI algorithms to accurately assess the DOA and improve real-time monitoring. Apart from BIS and EEG, other clinical signals have also been investigated to help monitor the DOA and other perioperative clinical data, which will be introduced in this chapter as well.

1 Application of AI in BIS

Artificial neural networks are commonly used in medical research to build prediction models. A multilayer feed-forward neural network was used to predict steady-state plasma drug concentration, which showed less prediction error than nonlinear mixed effects modeling (Brier et al. 1995). In a study of clinicians and artificial neural networks, researchers found the AI predicted a BIS value under 60 after bolus propofol injection better than clinicians with 10 common clinical parameters (Lin et al. 2002). Using spontaneous neuromuscular recovery and time elapsed since reversal, a simple feed-forward neural network predicted residual neuromuscular block (Laffey et al. 2003). As compared to traditional and statistical diagnostic models, feed-forward neural networks predicted postoperative nausea and vomiting (Peng et al. 2007), and hypotension (Lin et al. 2011) better. Additionally, artificial neural networks have been extensively used to interpret complicated data, such as electroencephalograms (EEGs). With a correlation coefficient of 0.94, a feed-forward neural network was trained to build a novel index of anesthesia depth based on raw EEG signals (Ortolani

B. Pei (✉)
Department of Anesthesiology, Shanghai Ninth People's Hospital, Shanghai Jiao Tong University School of Medicine, Shanghai, China

M. Xia, H. Jiang (eds.), *Artificial Intelligence in Anesthesiology*,
https://doi.org/10.1007/978-981-99-5925-9_4

et al. 2002). Preprocessed EEG was used to differentiate three anesthetic states using a recurrent neural network were capable of differentiating three anesthetic states using preprocessed EEG with an accuracy as high as 99.6% (Srinivasan et al. 2005). A feed-forward neural network model that combined preprocessed EEG with multiple vital signs to build a new DOA index was tested for prediction of anesthesia level, and the index showed less error and higher prediction accuracy than BIS (Sadrawi et al. 2015).

Traditionally, isobole and response surface models have been used to explain the pharmacodynamic interaction between propofol and remifentanil (Short et al. 2016; Bouillon et al. 2004). An empirical response surface model was recently used by Short et al. (2016) to predict the BIS value for propofol Ce and remifentanil Ce. There was a good correlation between predicted and measured BIS with a MDPE of 8 ± 24% and a MDAPE of 25 ± 13%. BIS prediction during propofol and remifentanil target-controlled infusions was better using artificial neural networks than traditional response surface models. Gambús et al. (2011) adopted a fuzzy logic-based artificial neural network (Adaptive Neuro-Fuzzy Inference System, ANFIS) to predict BIS from the combination of propofol Ce and remifentanil Ce during sedation-analgesia for endoscopic procedure. A validation group analysis found an MDPE of 5.83, MDAPE of 15.85, and RMSE of 13.25%, which is significantly less than the mistakes in the Short et al. (2016) study. As a result, the ANFIS model has been built using calculated Ce, which is inherently inaccurate in dynamic phases, and has only been tested in steady states. Induction and recovery periods of anesthesia may be less applicable to the ANFIS model. The use of feed-forward neural networks in combination with time series data may lead to enhanced predictive power in the dynamic phase due to the effective use of long and short-term memory to process time series data.

The empirical model aiming at optimizing data description has the disadvantage that it has no biological basis, and the parameters are difficult to interpret. Additionally, complex models with a large number of parameters are likely to exhibit overfitting, which decreases the predictive power of the empirical model. By using advanced computational methods such as deep learning, we addressed the weaknesses of empirical modeling by designing a model system that mimics the traditional mechanistic PK–PD model. This study contrasts substantially with the traditional PK model in terms of long- and short-term memory, as well as in terms of theoretical similarity. According to the traditional PK model, the change in drug amount over time in the final node of the long short-term memory is perfectly linear, as the previous time node affects the next time node. The study does not assume pharmacokinetic intermediaries such as plasma concentrations or Ce, which are sources of error in traditional PK–PD models, in our long short-term memory model. Based on the computation of the nonlinear dose–response relationship between propofol in the compartments and BIS measured in the chambers, a feed-forward neural network is the number of nodes in a feed-forward neural network with a hidden layer that can approximate any nonlinear function, unlike a simple feed-forward neural network that performs a similar task to multiple linear regression analysis layers (Hornik 1991). A hidden layer of the feed-forward neural network was used to estimate the effects of covariates and propofol and remifentanil combined. PD and PK parts were both fed covariates to improve performance, though PD was more error-prone than PK.

Its extensibility in various areas is the main advantage of Verotta's deep learning model architecture. Due to cost or ethical concerns, traditional PK–PD studies require frequent blood sampling and analysis of drug concentrations, which are major limitations. Verotta's study can perform more easily PK–PD studies in vulnerable subjects since the deep learning model only requires dosing history and measured effect. The second benefit of the deep learning model is that it can easily test the effects of multiple covariates. Because Verotta related covariates directly with effects rather than PK–PD parameters, the high-dimensionality problem associated with traditional covariate modeling can be eliminated (Verotta 2012). In the deep learning model, several covariates that affect propofol PK–PD can be quickly incorporated as input nodes (Upton et al. 1999; Johnson et al. 2004). These include cardiac output and hemorrhage. Another long short-term memory input can be used to model the combined effects of more than two drugs. Lastly, it is an excellent way to extend machine learning algorithms and software that are rapidly developing. Results of this study can also be applied clinically. Target-controlled infusion pumps can provide a BIS prediction curve to aid in determining the best dose of two synergistic drugs. By calculating the BIS from the input and node weights, deep learning can be applied immediately to target-controlled infusion devices, contrary to the learning process (Beam and Kohane 2016).

2 EEG with a Deep Learning Approach

In surgery, anesthetic drugs primarily affect the brain (Brambrink and Kirsch 2019). Physiological measures like blood pressure, heart rate, and blood oxygen level are usually used to measure the DOA during surgery. Patients and surgeries differ in these clinical parameters, depending on their age, body weight, gender, and medical history. Since vital signs are primary inputs in consciousness assessment, observing them is quite challenging. A BIS is used to reduce the incidence of awareness during total intravenous anesthesia by monitoring the effect of anesthetic agents by processing the online EEG. Commercial EEG monitors are known as BIS. Since BIS is still subject to patent access restrictions, it is not publicly available. In the BIS monitor, electrodes are molded onto the forehead to capture raw EEG signals and generate DOA scores ranging from 0 to 100 (Nimmo et al. 2019; Punjasawadwong et al. 2014). EEG-based DOA estimation is commonly performed using BIS.

EEG is a useful tool for recording brain activity and has been widely used to analyze and diagnose epilepsy, Alzheimer's disease, attention deficit hyperactivity disorder, and other disorders. As one of the common methods for monitoring, detecting, and diagnosing epilepsy, EEG measures the electrical activity of the brain through multiple electrodes placed at different locations in the brain, and the recorded signal usually contains multiple channels. Based on previous work, EEG signals are usually acquired by placing electrodes on the surface of the scalp or by short-term intracranial implantation, called scalp EEG and intracranial EEG, respectively. Although intracranial EEG recordings provide a better signal-to-noise ratio, intracranial electrodes have limited coverage and may miss discharges outside the coverage area, making them more demanding for the surgeon. Scalp EEG is a noninvasive technique that is more applicable and easy to use for daily patient monitoring and emergence alert generation.

There has been considerable progress in the use of machine learning methods in processing complex data, including deep learning (Ravì et al. 2016; Hong et al. 2020; Korkalainen et al. 2019). By creating a hybrid deep learning structure, this study attempts to mimic the BIS index online. EEG raw data is received by the network, and the DOA index is calculated without any handcrafted features elicited from the EEG. A deep neural network (DNN) outperforms feature-based classification systems as well as other DNN structures using large patient datasets (Bengio et al. 2013). A real-time forecast of continuous BIS scores is relatively new when used in the field of anesthesia. In this study, we combine deep learning methods in order to estimate the BIS index by using a regression model.

As deep learning is widely used and deeply promoted in the fields of image classification, natural language processing, and time series prediction, more and more deep learning models are proposed. In particular, deep learning algorithms possess the ability to learn high-level representations from natural signals (Mei et al. 2018), so it has achieved more prominent results in the medical field and signal processing. In EEG monitoring, deep learning models such as convolutional neural network (CNN) and stacked autoencoder (SAE) can learn feature representations directly from EEG data, thus replacing hand-designed feature extraction one way or another (Craley et al. 2021; Yang et al. 2020). The extracted features have been proven to be more robust and can achieve better performance detection.

BiLSTM networks have design advantages over CNNs in extracting temporal features of brain activities in different states one way or another, such as emotion recognition (Jia et al. 2020), motor imagery classification (Jin et al. 2018), and sleep staging (Lea et al. 2016). However, because information decays after many layers in the deep neural network structure, back propagation also leads to gradient disappearance problem when the long short-term memory (LSTM) network is faced with ultra-long sequences, which can weaken the reliability of the model. CNNs can extract displacement-invariant local patterns from input sequences as features for classification models, especially for learning features of multivariate time series data, e.g., for action or activity recognition (Morid et al. 2020), capturing hidden patterns of multivariate time series of healthcare data (Wang et al. 2019), and extracting period information for multivariate time series prediction (Yuan et al. 2017).

The DOA assessment has been proposed for a variety of features in a range of domains over the past few years. BIS indexes obtained using wavelet coefficient energy entropy and wavelet weighted median frequency, for instance, exhibit a high correlation with wavelets (Zoughi and Boostani 2010; Afrasiabi et al. 2012). A key feature of deep anesthesia detection is burst suppression. The nonlinear energy operator was used to detect and segment burst suppression automatically by Sarkela et al. (Särkelä et al. 2002) It is common for several studies to use sample entropy and permutation entropy features (Shalbaf et al. 2013, 2017; Liu et al. 2018). An important component of the BIS score is the instantaneous frequency (IF) (Lashkari and Boostani 2017). EEG can also be used to estimate the IF using a short-time Fourier transform. Moreover, Kalman filters are used to predict the cutoff frequencies of the band-pass filter through successive windows, resulting in a more accurate estimation of IF (Lashkari and Boostani 2017). It is possible to make decisions using various types of regressors and classifiers, such as artificial neural networks (Shalbaf et al. 2013), neuro-fuzzy inference systems with linguistic hedges (Shalbaf et al. 2017), and random forests (Liu et al. 2018). It is, however, mostly private datasets that are used in anesthesia research. DOA labels in datasets are assessed by anesthesiologists (Liu et al. 2019) or extracted from automatic EEG monitoring systems (Bengio et al. 2013; Liu et al. 2018).

Based on data collected from 231 subjects undergoing total intravenous anesthesia during surgery, Lee et al. (Bengio et al. 2013) developed a deep learning model. Besides the subject's characteristics, propofol, and remifentanil infusion histories are inputs into the network. By predicting continuous values, it determines the BIS score. Pharmacokinetic-pharmacodynamic model does not perform well in comparison to their developed method (Liu et al. 2019). Convolutional neural networks like CifarNet, AlexNet, and VGGNet are trained on the spectrograms of EEGs from 50 subjects. A big dataset requires computing intensive conversion of EEG signals into 2D images. A classification performance of 93.5% is achieved after only three levels of anesthesia, while it is more common to consider four anesthetized states before a classification is possible (Shalbaf et al. 2013, 2017; Liu et al. 2018). In Lee et al.'s study (Lee et al. 2019), a decision tree is built to classify BIS ranges using four parameters driven by the BIS monitor. BIS values are then calculated using multiple regression models. A dataset of 5427 subjects is being used to train the model. As compared to our end-to-end deep learning model, this method is less generalized and more susceptible to noise.

Most feature-based methods combine expert handcrafted features with classifiers that focus more on extracting handcrafted features from background patterns, and common features include time-domain methods, frequency-domain methods, time-frequency-domain methods, and nonlinear methods. Classifiers often use traditional machine learning methods.

However, in many fields, features extracted by deep learning methods are more robust than handcrafted features. In the literature (Truong et al. 2018), the short-time Fourier transform (STFT) was used to extract the time and frequency domain information of EEG signals, and a CNN architecture consisting of three blocks (each block includes a normalization layer, a convolutional layer, and a maximum pooling layer) was used for feature extraction and classification. In the literature (Ullah et al. 2018), instead of feature extraction for EEG signals, a pyramidal one-dimensional deep convolutional neural network was directly used to detect single-channel EEG signals, and the experimental results showed that CNNs learn better than manual engineering techniques.

Manual feature extraction requires a large amount of domain knowledge, and selecting only some EEG channels will lose some useful information. Although EEG signals are usually dynamic and nonlinear, the signals can be considered smooth over sufficiently small time periods. Different brain regions may have different effects on epilepsy, different brain regions have different EEG data characteristics for epilepsy, and there may be local dependence between different channels. The characteristics of EEG signals at one point in time have different degrees of correlation with data from past time points and data from future time points. In contrast, in the field of natural language processing, self-attentive mechanisms are often used to capture contextual relationships. For example, the literature (Li et al. 2020) proposes a BiLSTM model with a self-attentive mechanism and multi-channel features, which combines multiple feature vectors and the implicit output of the BiLSTM model to give different sentiment weights to different words using the self-attentive mechanism. It can effectively improve the importance of sentiment polar words and fully exploit the sentiment information in the text. A Chinese-named entity recognition model based on multi-scale local contextual features and self-attentiveness mechanism is proposed in the literature (Guo et al. 2020). The original bidirectional long short-term memory and conditional random field (BiLSTM-CRF) model is modified by fusing convolutional neural networks (CNNs) with different kernel sizes to extract multi-scale local contextual features. The self-attentive mechanism breaks the limitation of BiLSTM-CRF in capturing process dependencies, and further improves the performance of the model.

EEG as a key technology for brain–computer interface can be divided into five stages in terms of its application method (Ilyas et al. 2015). The first stage is the acquisition of EEG signals. The second stage is the preprocessing of EEG signals, which aims to remove noise interference. The original EEG signal contains interfering signals of eye, heart, and muscle, and removing the interfering signals can simplify the subsequent analysis and processing of EEG signals. The third stage is EEG signal feature extraction. The features are extracted from the preprocessed EEG signals to distinguish different EEG signals, and to reduce the dimensionality of the signals to simplify the calculation process. The fourth stage is the classification of the extracted features. The selection of the appropriate classifier is an important factor affecting the classification effect. The fifth stage is to use the classification results for the control of external devices or to give judgment results. Preprocessing, feature extraction, and classification of EEG signals are important elements of EEG signal processing and have been widely and deeply studied (Motamedi-Fakhr et al. 2014; Tambe and Khachane 2016).

The raw EEG signal contains eye, ECG, EMG, and other noises, and also industrial frequency interference is an important source of EEG artifacts, which increase the complexity of EEG signal processing and increase the amount of operations during processing, and need to be stripped before signal analysis (Rajya Lakshmi et al. 2014). The main EEG signal preprocessing methods are Common Spatial Patterns (CSP), Principal Components Analysis (PCA), Common Average Referencing (CAR), adaptive filtering, Independent Component Analysis (ICA), Digital Filter, etc.

After preprocessing, the original EEG signal becomes a relatively pure EEG signal with various artifacts and noise removed, but due to the large amount of EEG signal data, direct processing is too complicated, and feature extraction is needed to reduce the dimensionality of the data (Ilyas et al. 2015). At present, the commonly used signal feature extraction methods are Power

Spectrum Density (PSD), Principal Component Analysis (PCA), Independent Component Analysis (ICA), Auto Regressive Analysis (AR), Wavelet Transform (WT), Wavelet Packet Transform (WPT), Fast Fourier Transform (FFT), etc.

After the EEG signal is preprocessed and feature extracted, the extracted feature vectors are classified by classifier to achieve the analysis and prediction of EEG signal. Commonly used EEG signal classifiers include k-Nearest Neighbor (k-NN), Linear Discriminant Analysis (LDA), Support Vector Machine (SVM), Naive Bayes (NB), Artificial Neural Network (ANN), and Deep Learning (DL).

2.1 Common Spatial Patterns

The common spatial pattern (CSP) in signal processing is a mathematical method for separating multivariate signals into additive subcomponents that have the largest variance difference between two windows. CSP filtering is derived from Common Spatial Subspace Decomposition (CSSD), the basic idea of CSSD algorithm is to find a direction in the high-dimensional space that maximizes the variance of one class while minimizing the variance of the other class when classifying two cases. The basic idea is to design a spatial filter to process the EEG signal to obtain a new time series that maximizes the variance of one type of signal while minimizing the variance of the other type of signal, thus obtaining the feature with the largest variance. The advantage of this algorithm is that it does not require pre-selection of specific frequency bands, but the disadvantage is that it is noise sensitive and depends on multi-channel analysis (Pei and Yang 2018).

2.2 Principal Component Analysis

PCA is the process of computing the principal components and using them to perform a change of basis on the data, sometimes using only the first few principal components and ignoring the rest. It is a statistical method that transforms a set of correlated independent variables into linearly uncorrelated variables through an orthogonal transformation, and the transformed variables are called "principal components." The function of principal component analysis is to reduce the dimensionality of vectors and the complexity of signal feature extraction and classification. In EEG signal processing applications, principal component analysis decomposes the EEG signal into uncorrelated components with maximum variance, separates the interfering components with large amplitude such as EEG and EMG, and then reconstructs the EEG signal to achieve signal denoising (Liu and Yao 2006).

2.3 Common Average Reference

CAR is a computationally simple technique, and therefore amenable to both on-chip and real-time applications.

2.4 Adaptive Filter

The adaptive filter comprises a linear filter with variable parameters and a method to adjust each parameter according to an optimization algorithm. In most cases, adaptive filters are digital filters due to the complexity of optimization algorithms. It is a filter that automatically adjusts its parameters without knowing the statistical characteristics of the input signal and noise in advance, and gradually estimates the desired statistical characteristics during operation to adjust its own parameters to achieve the best filtering effect. A complete adaptive filter consists of four main parts: the input signal, the reference signal, the filter, and the parameter adjustment.

2.5 Independent Component Analysis

An independent component analysis (ICA) involves separating multivariate signals into additive subcomponents as part of signal processing. It is a blind source analysis method that separates artifacts from the EEG signal as independent components based on data characteristics. According to the theory of ICA algorithm, oculomotor artifacts, ECG artifacts, EMG artifacts, and IDF interferences are generated by independent sources with statistical independence, which can be separated by the ICA algorithm to extract useful EEG signals. ICA algorithm provides an effective method for separating and removing oculomotor artifacts from EEG signals, and Matthew B. Pontifex et al. explored a fully automated ICA component separation method for eye-movement artifacts that avoids mis-segregation of signal components resembling the distribution of eye-movement artifacts in scalp EEG and reduces the potential for human error in identifying artifacts (Pontifex et al. 2017a). In the same year in the same journal, Matthew B. Pontifex et al. also explored the possibility that the variability associated with the uncertainty of the ICA algorithm may affect the reconstruction of the EEG signal after the removal of the oculomotor artifact component. Matthew B. Pontifex et al. performed ICA analysis of EEG signal data from 32 university students using three different ICA algorithms repeated 30 times. The results showed that the ICA algorithm may introduce other artifacts in the reconstruction of EEG signals after removing artifact components, and careful selection of the ICA algorithm and parameters may reduce this effect (Pontifex et al. 2017b).

2.6 Power Spectrum Density

Power spectral density defines how the power of a time series signal is distributed with frequency and is a probability statistic that is a measure of the mean square value of a random variable. The results showed that there were statistically significant differences between the "between" and "before" and "after" periods. The results show that there are statistical differences between the "interphase" and "before" and "after" periods, and that the fractal dimensions are also significantly different, and that these differences help to understand the changes in the sleep fusiform waves (De Dea et al. 2018).

2.7 Auto Regressive Analysis

AR analysis is a time-domain analysis method for feature extraction by fitting EEG signal data with a mathematical model. AR models can be formulated as linear prediction problems, where for time series data, the predicted value at the current point can be approximated by a linear weighted sum of the sampled values of the n closest previous points. AR models commonly used in EEG signal analysis can be further classified into adaptive and non-adaptive models (Li et al. 2009).

2.8 Wavelet Transform and Wavelet Packet Transform

Wavelet transform is a time-frequency transform method, which inherits and develops the idea of localization of short-time Fourier transform, and can provide a "time-frequency" window that changes with frequency. The wavelet transform highlights the signal characteristics and refines the signal at multiple scales through the telescopic translation operation to achieve higher time resolution at high frequencies and higher frequency resolution at low frequencies, which automatically adapts to the requirements of signal time-frequency analysis. The wavelet transform decomposes only the low-frequency part of the signal, but not the high-frequency part, so the frequency resolution decreases as the signal frequency increases. The discrete wavelet transform (DWT) of EEG signals from migraine patients was performed, and 23 feature quantities were extracted from each channel signal, and all of them were used for pattern recognition after secondary screening (Subasi et al. 2019). The quality factor Q of the discrete wavelet transform wavelet basis function is fixed, while the quality factor Q of the Tunable Q-factor Wavelet Transform (TQWT) is adjustable to adjust the wavelet oscillation characteristics to match the characteristic waveform oscillation characteristics. TQWT generally decomposes EEG signals into different sub-bands based on the quality factor Q, redundancy R, and the number of decomposition layers J. Because of the random non-smooth characteristics of EEG signals, the quality factor Q takes a larger value, for example, Q takes 14 (Al Ghayab et al. 2019). Wavelet packet transform has a higher resolution than wavelet transform for high-frequency signals and is a more refined analysis method, which is used for feature extraction in studies based on EEG signals such as lie detection, facial expression recognition, driving intention recognition, etc., to obtain better classification results (Dodia et al. 2019; Edla et al. 2018; Li et al. 2018).

2.9 Fast Fourier Transform

Fast Fourier Transform is a fast algorithm of discrete Fourier Transform, and in EEG signal feature extraction, FFT transforms EEG signal from the time domain to frequency domain and does spectral analysis or calculates power spectral density. FFT is also used for fatigue driving EEG signal analysis and driver EEG signal analysis in unmanned driving system driving behavior simulation experiments (Dkhil et al. 2018; Yang and Ma 2018).

EEG signal feature extraction is an important step in EEG signal classification and recognition, EEG signal is the superposition of potentials formed by various electrophysiological activities of the brain on the surface of the scalp, which has random and non-smooth characteristics, how to extract useful features from the complex EEG signal is the key to EEG signal analysis. The band-pass filtering of the EEG signal according to its frequency distribution is not sufficient to reflect its characteristics, and the high-dimensional feature vector will bring a very complex operation to the subsequent classification algorithm, so it is necessary to do the dimensionality reduction process, generally using PCA or ICA dimensionality reduction.

2.10 Linear Discriminant Analysis

LDA is a linear learning method proposed by Fisher in 1936. The main idea of LDA is: for a given set of training samples, find the appropriate projection direction to project the samples onto a straight line, so that the projection points of the same class are concentrated as much as possible and the projection points of different classes are as far away as possible (Zhou 2016). LDA is not too computationally intensive, easy to use, and is a good classification method.

2.11 Support Vector Machine

The basic principle of SVM is to find the optimal decision surface in space so that different classes of data can be distributed on both sides of the decision surface to achieve classification (Li 2018). Siuly et al. performed the optimum allocation based principal component analysis method (OA_PCA) for feature extraction and tested four popular classifiers: least square support vector machine (LS-SVM), naive bayes classifier (NB), k-nearest neighbor algorithm (KNN), and linear discriminant analysis (LDA). The results showed that the classification accuracy of LS-SVM was up to 100%, which was 7.10% more accurate than the existing classification algorithms for epilepsy EEG data (Siuly and Li 2015).

2.12 Naive Bayes

The Naive Bayesian classifier is a simple and practical classifier based on Bayes' theorem, and in some fields its efficiency is comparable to that of some other classifiers (Tahernezhad-Javazm et al. 2018; Machado and Balbinot 2014; Mehmood et al. 2017). The main idea of the Naive Bayesian is that for a given item to be classified, solve for the probability of occurrence of each category under the conditions of this item's occurrence, and whichever category is the largest, the item to be classified belongs to that category. The Naive Bayesian algorithm assumes that the samples are independent of each other and uncorrelated (Obeidat and Mansour 2018). The Naive Bayesian classifier has outstanding features of speed, efficiency, and simple algorithm structure when used to process high-dimensional data (Katkar and Kulkarni 2013). Based on the Naive Bayesian algorithm researchers have proposed various improved algorithms, such as tree augmented Naive Bayesian algorithm and network augmented plain Bayesian algorithm, which all aim to improve the algorithm performance and increase the classification accuracy (Tahernezhad-Javazm et al. 2018).

2.13 Artificial Neural Network

ANN is a hot research topic in the field of AI since the 1980s, which abstracts the neuronal network of human brain from the perspective of information processing and builds corresponding models to form different networks with different connection methods. It is a branch of machine learning methods.

ANN is widely used in the field of medical diagnosis, especially in the detection and analysis of biomedical signals, and can be used to solve problems that are difficult or impossible to solve by conventional methods in biomedical signal processing, and has been widely used in EEG, ECG, oncology, and psychiatry (Dande and Samant 2018; Ventouras et al. 2005). Payal Dande et al. present a trained and learned ANN for the diagnosis of tuberculosis with a sensitivity and specificity of 100% and 72% (Dande and Samant 2018), respectively. Enzo Grossi et al. used an ANN-based MS-ROM/I-FAST system to extract features of interest from EEG for the differential diagnosis of autism in children with good results, requiring only a few minutes of EEG data and without any data preprocessing (Grossi et al. 2017).

References

Afrasiabi S, Boostani R, Koochaki S, Zand F. Presenting an effective EEG-based index to monitor the depth of anesthesia. In: The 16th CSI Int. symposium on artificial intelligence and signal processing (AISP 2012). IEEE; 2012. p. 557–62.

Al Ghayab HR, Yan Li S, Siuly SA. A feature extraction technique based on tunable Q-factor wavelet transform for brain signal classification. J Neurosci Methods. 2019;312:43–52.

Beam AL, Kohane IS. Translating artificial intelligence into clinical care. JAMA. 2016;316:2368–9.

Bengio Y, Courville A, Vincent P. Representation learning: a review and new perspectives. IEEE Trans Pattern Anal Mach Intell. 2013;35(8):1798–828.

Bouillon TW, Bruhn J, Radulescu L, Andresen C, Shafer TJ, Cohane C, Shafer SL. Pharmacodynamic interaction between propofol and remifentanil regarding hypnosis, tolerance of laryngoscopy, bispectral index, and electroencephalographic approximate entropy. Anesthesiology. 2004;100:1353–72.

Brambrink AM, Kirsch JR. Essentials of neurosurgical anesthesia & critical care: strategies for prevention, early detection, and successful management of perioperative complications. Springer Nature; 2019.

Brier ME, Zurada JM, Aronoff GR. Neural network predicted peak and trough gentamicin concentrations. Pharm Res. 1995;12:406–12.

Craley J, Johnson E, Jouny C, et al. Automated interpatient seizure detection using multichannel convolutional and recurrent neural networks. Biomed Signal Process Control. 2021;64:102360.

Dande P, Samant P. Acquaintance to artificial neural networks and use of artificial intelligence as a diagnostic tool for tuberculosis: a review. Tuberculosis. 2018;108:1–9.

De Dea F, Zanus C, Carrozzi M. Power spectral density analysis in spindles epochs in healthy children. In: World congress on medical physics and biomedical engineering; 2018. p. 247–51.

Dkhil MB, Wali A, Alimi AM. Drowsy driver detection by EEG analysis using fast Fourier transform. In: Electrical engineering and systems science; 2018.

Dodia S, Edla DR, et al. An efficient EEG based deceit identification test using wavelet packet transform and linear discriminant analysis. J Neurosci Methods. 2019;314:31–40.

Edla DR, Ansari MF, et al. Classification of facial expressions from EEG signals using wavelet packet transform and SVM for wheelchair control operations. Procedia Comput Sci. 2018;132:1467–76.

Gambús PL, Jensen EW, Jospin M, Borrat X, Martínez Pallí G, Fernández-Candil J, Valencia JF, Barba X, Caminal P, Trocóniz IF. Modeling the effect of propofol and remifentanil combinations for sedation-analgesia in endoscopic procedures using an adaptive neuro fuzzy inference system (ANFIS). Anesth Analg. 2011;112:331–9.

Grossi E, Olivieri C, Buscema M. Diagnosis of autism through EEG processed by advanced computational algorithms: a pilot study. Comput Methods Prog Biomed. 2017;142:73–9.

Guo X, Zhou H, Su J, et al. Chinese agricultural diseases and pests named entity recognition with multi-scale

local context features and self-attention mechanism. Comput Electron Agric. 2020;179:105830.
Hong S, Zhou Y, Shang J, Xiao C, Sun J. Opportunities and challenges of deep learning methods for electrocardiogram data: a systematic review. Comput Biol Med. 2020;122:103801.
Hornik K. Approximation capabilities of multilayer feedforward networks. Neural Netw. 1991;4: 251–7.
Ilyas MZ, Saad P, Ahmad MI. A survey of analysis and classification of EEG signals for brain-computer interfaces. 2015 2nd international conference on biomedical engineering(ICoBE). Penang; 2015.
Jia ZY, Lin YF, Liu TH, et al. Motor imagery classification based on multiscale feature extraction and squeeze-excitation model. J Comput Res Dev. 2020;57(12):2481–9.
Jin HH, Yin HB, He LN. Deep automatic sleep staging model using synthetic minority technique. J Comput Appl. 2018;38(9):2483–8.
Johnson KB, Egan TD, Kern SE, McJames SW, Cluff ML, Pace NL. Influence of hemorrhagic shock followed by crystalloid resuscitation on propofol: a pharmacokinetic and pharmacodynamic analysis. Anesthesiology. 2004;101:647–59.
Katkar MVD, Kulkarni MSV. A novel parallel implementation of naive Bayesian classifier for big data; 2013. International Conference on Green Computing, Communication and Conservation of Energy (IEEE). p. 847–52.
Korkalainen H, Aakko J, Nikkonen S, Kainulainen S, Leino A, Duce B, Afara IO, Myllymaa S, Töyräs J, Leppänen T. Accurate deep learning-based sleep staging in a clinical population with suspected obstructive sleep apnea. IEEE J Biomed Health Inform. 2019;24(7):2073–81.
Laffey JG, Tobin E, Boylan JF, McShane AJ. Assessment of a simple artificial neural network for predicting residual neuromuscular block. Br J Anaesth. 2003;90:48–52.
Lashkari A, Boostani R. A kalman-based instantaneous frequency estimation for anesthetic depth measurement. In: 2017 22nd Int. Conf. On digital signal processing (DSP). IEEE; 2017. p. 1–4.
Lea C, Vidal R, Reiter A, et al. Temporal convolutional networks: a unified approach to action segmentation[C]// ECCV 2016: Computer vision – ECCV 2016 workshops, Amsterdam, Oct 8-10 and 15-16, 2016. Berlin, Heidelberg: Springer; 2016. p. 47–54.
Lee H-C, Ryu H-G, Park Y, Yoon SB, Yang SM, Oh H-W, Jung C-W. Data driven investigation of bispectral index algorithm. Sci Rep. 2019;9(1):1–8.
Li Y. Recognition algorithm of driving fatigue related problems based on EEG signals. NeuroQuantology. 2018;16(6):517–23.
Li Y, Qiu Y, Zhu Y. EEG signal analysis methods and their applications [M]. Science Press; 2009.
Min Li, Wuhong Wang, et al. Identification of driving intention based on EEG signals. J Bei Institute Technol 2018, 27(3): 357–362.
Li W, Qi F, Tang M, et al. Bidirectional LSTM with self-attention mechanism and multi-channel features for sentiment classification. Neurocomputing. 2020;387:63–77.
Lin C-S, Li Y-C, Mok MS, Wu C-C, Chiu H-W, Lin Y-H. Neural network modeling to predict the hypnotic effect of propofol bolus induction. Amia. 2002;2002:450–3.
Lin CS, Chang CC, Chiu JS, Lee YW, Lin JA, Mok MS, Chiu HW, Li YC. Application of an artificial neural network to predict postinduction hypotension during general anesthesia. Med Decis Mak. 2011;31:308–14.
Liu T, Yao D. Removal of the ocular artifacts from EEG data using a cascaded spatio-temporal processing. Comput Methods Programs Biomed. 2006;83:95–103.
Liu Q, Ma L, Fan S-Z, Abbod MF, Shieh J-S. Sample entropy analysis for the estimating depth of anaesthesia through human EEG signal at different levels of unconsciousness during surgeries. Peer J. 2018;6:e4817.
Liu Q, Cai J, Fan S-Z, Abbod MF, Shieh J-S, Kung Y, Lin L. Spectrum analysis of EEG signals using CNN to model patient's consciousness level based on anesthesiologists' experience, vol. 7. IEEE Access; 2019. p. 53 731–42.
Machado J, Balbinot A. Executed movement using EEG signals through a naive Bayes classifier. Micromachines. 2014;5:1082–105.
Mehmood RM, Du R, Lee HJ. Optimal feature selection and deep learning ensembles method for emotion recognition from human brain EEG sensors. Digital Object Identifier. 2017;5. 10.1109/ACCESS:2724555.
Mei ZN, Zhao X, Chen HY, et al. Bio-signal complexity analysis in epileptic seizure monitoring: a topic review. Sensors. 2018;18(6):1720.
Morid MA, Sheng ORL, Kawamoto K, et al. Learning hidden patterns from patient multivariate time series data using convolutional neural networks: a case study of healthcare cost prediction. J Biomed Inform. 2020;111:103565.
Motamedi-Fakhr S, Moshrefi-Torbati M, et al. Signal processing techniques applied to human sleep EEG signals-a review. Biomed Signal Process Control. 2014;10:21–33.
Nimmo A, Absalom A, Bagshaw O, Biswas A, Cook T, Costello A, Grimes S, Mulvey D, Shinde S, Whitehouse T, et al. Guidelines for the safe practice of total intravenous anaesthesia (TIVA) joint guidelines from the association of anaesthetists and the society for intravenous anaesthesia. Anaesthesia. 2019;74(2):211–24.
Obeidat DRMA, Mansour DRAM. EEG based epilepsy diagnosis system using reconstruction phase space and naive Bayes classifier. In: Wseas transactions on circuits and systems, vol. 17; 2018. p. 159–68.
Ortolani O, Conti A, Di Filippo A, Adembri C, Moraldi E, Evangelisti A, Maggini M, Roberts SJ. EEG signal processing in anaesthesia: use of a neural network technique for monitoring depth of anaesthesia. Br J Anaesth. 2002;88:644–8.

Pei Y, Yang S. Advances in motor imagery EEG signal algorithm research. Beijing Biomed Eng. 2018;37(2):208–14.

Peng SY, Wu KC, Wang JJ, Chuang JH, Peng SK, Lai YH. Predicting postoperative nausea and vomiting with the application of an artificial neural network. Br J Anaesth. 2007;98:60–5.

Pontifex MB, Miskovic V, Laszlo S. Evaluating the efficacy of fully automated approaches for the selection of eyeblink ICA components. Psychophysiology. 2017a;54:780–91.

Pontifex MB, Gwizdala KL, Parks AC, Billinger M, Brunner C. Variability of ICA decomposition may impact EEG signals when used to remove eyeblink artifacts. Psychophysiology. 2017b;54:386–98.

Punjasawadwong Y, Phongchiewboon A, Bunchungmongkol N. Bispectral index for improving anaesthetic delivery and postoperative recovery. Cochrane Database Syst Rev. 2014;214(6):CD003843.

Rajya Lakshmi M, Dr TV, Prasad D, Chandra Prakash V. Survey on EEG signal processing methods. Int J Adv Res Comput Sci Softw Eng. 2014;4:84–91.

Ravì D, Wong C, Deligianni F, Berthelot M, Andreu-Perez J, Lo B, Yang G-Z. Deep learning for health informatics. IEEE J Biomed Health Inform. 2016;21(1):4–21.

Sadrawi M, Fan SZ, Abbod MF, Jen KK, Shieh JS. Computational depth of anesthesia via multiple vital signs based on artificial neural networks. Biomed Res Int. 2015;2015:536863.

Särkelä M, Mustola S, Seppänen T, Koskinen M, Lepola P, Suominen K, Juvonen T, Tolvanen-Laakso H, Jäntti V. Automatic analysis and monitoring of burst suppression in anesthesia. J Clin Monit Comput. 2002;17(2):125–34.

Shalbaf R, Behnam H, Sleigh JW, Steyn-Ross A, Voss LJ. Monitoring the depth of anesthesia using entropy features and an artificial neural network. J Neurosci Methods. 2013;218(1):17–24.

Shalbaf A, Saffar M, Sleigh JW, Shalbaf R. Monitoring the depth of anesthesia using a new adaptive neurofuzzy system. IEEE J Biomed Health Inform. 2017;22(3):671–7.

Short TG, Hannam JA, Laurent S, Campbell D, Misur M, Merry AF, Tam YH. Refining target-controlled infusion: an assessment of pharmacodynamic target-controlled infusion of propofol and remifentanil using a response surface model of their combined effects on bispectral index. Anesth Analg. 2016;122:90–7.

Siuly S, Li Y. Designing a robust feature extraction method based on optimum allocation and principal component analysis for epileptic EEG signal classification. Comput Methods Programs Biomed. 2015;119:29–42.

Srinivasan V, Eswaran C, Sriraam N. EEG based automated detection of anesthetic levels using a recurrent artificial neural network. Int J Bioelectromagn. 2005;7:267–70.

Subasi A, Ahmed A, et al. Effect of photic stimulation for migraine detection using random forest and discrete wavelet transform. Biomed Signal Process Control. 2019;49:231–9.

Tahernezhad-Javazm F, Azimirad V, Shoaran M. A review and experimental study on the application of classifiers and evolutionary algorithms in EEG-based brain–machine interface systems. J Neural Eng. 2018;15:021007. (39 pp).

Namita R. Tambe, Ajitkumar Khachane. Mood based E-learning using EEG. 2nd international conference on computing, communication, control and automation, 2016.

Truong ND, Nguyen AD, Kuhlmann L, et al. Convolutional neural networks for seizure prediction using intracranial and scalp electroencephalogram. Neural Netw. 2018;105:104–11.

Ullah I, Hussain M, Qazi E-U-H, et al. An automated system for epilepsy detection using EEG brain signals based on deep learning approach. Expert Syst Appl. 2018;107:61–71.

Upton RN, Ludbrook GL, Grant C, Martinez AM. Cardiac output is a determinant of the initial concentrations of propofol after short-infusion administration. Anesth Analg. 1999;89:545–52.

Ventouras EM, Monoyiou EA, Ktonas PY, Paparrigopoulos T, Dikeos DG, Uzunoglu NK, Soldatos CR. Sleep spindle detection using artificial neural networks trained with filtered time-domain EEG: a feasibility study. Comput Methods Prog Biomed. 2005;78:191–207.

Verotta D. Covariate modeling in population PK/PD models: an open problem. Adv Pharmacoepidem Drug Safety. 2012;S1:006.

Wang K, Li K, Zhou L, et al. Multiple convolutional neural networks for multivariate time series prediction. Neurocomputing. 2019;360:107–19.

Yang L, Ma R. Driving behavior recognition using EEG data from a simulated car-following experiment. Accid Anal Prev. 2018;116:30–40.

Yang J, Huang X, Wu H, et al. EEG-based emotion classification based on bidirectional long short-term memory network. Procedia Comput Sci. 2020;174:491–504.

Yuan Y, Xun GX, Jia KB, et al. A multi-view deep learning method for epileptic seizure detection using short-time Fourier transform[C]//ACM-BCB'17: proceedings of the 8th ACM international conference on bioinformatics, computational biology, and health informatics, Boston, Aug 20-23, 2017. New York: Association for Computing Machinery; 2017. p. 213–22.

Zhou Z. Machine learning [M]. Tsinghua University Publishing House Co., Ltd; 2016.

Zoughi T, Boostani R. Presenting a combinatorial feature to estimate depth of anesthesia. Int J Signal Process. 2010;6(2):10–4.

Artificial Intelligence in Airway Management

Ming Xia

Airway management is anesthetists' main task during a surgical procedure, which crosses through the whole perioperative period—from the preoperative airway assessment to the postoperative management in SICU. This chapter introduces the ways in which AI techniques are applied in different steps of the airway management process, namely the assessment, induction, maintenance, and management after the surgery, especially when encountering difficult airways during these steps. Related techniques include face recognition analysis, speech features analysis, and support vector machine. These methods integrating AI techniques are featured with higher sensitivity and specificity, which defines their prospective future development in the airway field.

1 AI in Prediction of Difficult Airway

Prediction of a difficult airway is an essential part of preoperative assessment since difficult airway management has always been one of the main causes of adverse events related to anesthesia, especially oral anesthesia, and has the potential to cause life-threatening complications. Thus, the prediction of difficult airways before surgery has been a topic of concern for anesthesiologists.

An analysis of claims related to airway management in the UK (Cook and Macdougall-Davis 2012) and the USA (Metzner et al. 2011) shows that respiratory events, such as difficult intubation and inadequate ventilation, are the leading causes of poor clinical outcomes (severe harm, brain damage, and death). When the patient is not able to breathe with a face mask or be intubated with an endotracheal tube, the worst-case scenario in airway management arises. A similar situation is estimated to occur between 0.01 and 3 in 10,000 people (Heard et al. 2009). The inability to either ventilate or intubate is the most common cause of death attributed to anesthesia in modern times (Hove et al. 2007). The advancement of laryngoscopy and monitoring of the placement of endotracheal tubes has allowed ease of intubations (Aziz et al. 2011; Teoh et al. 2010; Serocki et al. 2010), but difficult intubations remain a concern (Cook and Macdougall-Davis 2012).

Preoperative detection and prediction of a difficult airway are essential to patient safety. It is recommended that specific equipment and personnel be called in if there is a reasonable possibility of difficulty during intubation. Bedside tests are commonly used by anesthesiologists to predict the difficulty of tracheal intubations, but they have a low correlation with actual results.

M. Xia (✉)
Department of Anesthesiology, Shanghai Ninth People's Hospital, Shanghai Jiao Tong University School of Medicine, Shanghai, China
e-mail: xiaming1980@xzhmu.edu.cn

M. Xia, H. Jiang (eds.), *Artificial Intelligence in Anesthesiology*,
https://doi.org/10.1007/978-981-99-5925-9_5

Besides using existing bedside tests, experienced anesthesiologists should make more comprehensive clinical judgments based on morphologic parameters. However, even with fine-tuned preoperative airway assessments, some difficult airway patients are still not identified.

Based on the traditional methods, there are prediction techniques with the application of AI being developed, mainly techniques integrating facial analysis techniques and speech features analysis techniques. These methods mainly acquire parameters that are also acquired in traditional methods, and analyze them with a developed model or algorithm. In this way, the analysis could be in an automated and a faster manner, and at the same time, the specificity and efficacy of the prediction are raised.

In the following sections, AI techniques used in difficult airway prediction will be introduced in a more detailed way.

1.1 Facial Analysis Techniques in Difficult Airway Prediction

In areas such as marketing and emotion analysis (Ahn and Picard 2014; Ringeval et al. 2014), face recognition systems to improve vehicle safety (Dong et al. 2009; Gao et al. 2014) as well as in medicine (Baynam et al. 2011; Claes et al. 2012; Zhao et al. 2013; Zhu and Ramanan 2012), computer vision methods are being used extensively. A fast and robust face recognizer can now be built using facial landmark detection and tracking (Cevikalp et al. 2013; Xiong and De La Torre 2013). Those can detect and interpret specific features of the face, based on landmark positions, making them suitable for facial morphology analysis.

An automated method for predicting the difficult airway has been developed by Gabriel Louis Cuendet et al. (2016a). An algorithmic model was built using artificial intelligence (AI) to predict difficult airways using face data from a patient database and facial feature points fitted according to an algorithm. It had the same level of accuracy as manual assessment of difficult airways based on ROC validation. With a simple facial scan alone, this study provides an idea for the development of a more convenient and intelligent prediction model for difficult airways. This study's small sample size requires further investigation and validation of the face scanning prediction method for difficult airways.

A deep learning model was designed by Hayasaka et al. (2021) for predicting intubation difficulty. Study participants excluded those undergoing surgery with altered facial appearance, surgery with altered neck range of motion, or intubation performed by a physician with less than 3 years of anesthesia experience at Yamagata University Hospital. The patients were photographed 16 times after surgery. A deep learning classification model was developed by linking the patient's facial image with the difficulty of intubation, and all images were categorized as "easy" or "difficult" by an anesthesiologist. Intuiting a real patient and developing an AI model led to the development of receiver operating characteristic curves (ROC curves) with sensitivity, specificity, and area under the curve (AUC) being calculated; median AUC was used. The AI model's classification of intubation difficulties was visualized using class activation heat maps. Supine-side, mouth-base-closed images were used to generate the most accurate AI model for classifying intubation difficulties. As a result, 80.5% accuracy, 81.8% sensitivity, 83.3% specificity, 0.864 AUC, and 95% confidence interval [0.731–0.969], indicating a significant concentration of class activation thermograms around the neck, regardless of the background. AI identifies intubation difficulties by recognizing facial contours. This study is the first to use deep learning (CNN) for the classification of intubation difficulties. The AI model developed in this study may be useful for inexperienced medical personnel performing tracheal intubation under general anesthesia or in emergency situations.

Based on the two studies mentioned above, it is not difficult to come to the conclusion that the prediction of difficult airway with AI are actually based on traditional prediction methods.

The Mallampati score assesses the airway according to the visibility of oropharyngeal structures observed on a sitting patient with the mouth wide open and the tongue out. The author suggests that the larger the base of the tongue, the more it overshadows the larynx, resulting in a poor laryngoscopic view and a potentially difficult laryngoscopy. Endotracheal intubation difficulty can therefore be assessed by the volume of the tongue, which is a difficult parameter to measure. The tongue's volume cannot be determined in relation to the capacity of the oropharyngeal cavity, so it makes sense that the base of the tongue is disproportionately large when it can mask the visibility of the facial pillars and uvula. Depending on the score, the oropharyngeal structure is either fully visible or not visible. Mallampati and modified Mallampati tests reported varying sensitivity and specificity. Based on the report of Cattano et al. (2004), sensitivity and specificity were reported at 35% and 91%, respectively. Lundstrøm et al. (2011) included 55 studies and 177,088 patients, and reported a sensitivity of 0–100% and a specificity of 44–100%. Based on ROC analysis, the diagnostic test was classified as good when the area under the curve (AUC) was 0.753. There was a report by Lee et al. (2006) that the AUC of the Mallampati test and the modified Mallampati test was 0.58 and 0.83, respectively. As the Mallampati test does not have significant discriminatory power when used alone, its clinical value is limited.

By moving the lower jaw forward (in a movement of prognathism), Khan et al. (2003) evaluated the patient's ability to cover his upper lip with his lower incisors. In grades I and II, laryngoscopy is predicted to be easy, and in grades III, it is predicted to be difficult. There was an initial sensitivity of 76.5% and a specificity of 88.7% reported by the authors. Recently, those results were confirmed by 78.95% and 91.96% of participants in a study (Khan et al. 2009).

A study performed by Eberhart et al. (2005) compared Mallampati score with upper lip bite test as a preoperative bedside screening test for difficult laryngoscopy and concluded that both tests provided poor preoperative predictions of difficult laryngoscopy. Airway management problems cannot be predicted by any of those simple tests. Predicting difficult endotracheal intubations is generally difficult due to their low sensitivity and predictive positive values. A multivariate analysis score has thus been proposed in several studies.

The thyromental distance (TMD) is also called the Patil-Aldreti test, it measures the distance from the upper edge of the thyroid cartilage to the chin when the patient's head is fully extended. When TMD is short, it means that the anterior lying larynx is at a more acute angle. It also equates a less space for the tongue to be compressed when using the laryngoscope. A thyromental distance greater than 7 cm is usually associated with easy intubation whereas a thyromental distance smaller than 6 cm may predict a difficult intubation. This predictor itself is not a good predictor for difficult intubation because of its low sensitivity and specificity (48% and 70%) (Baker et al. 2009), which obliges its combination with other methods. The ratio of height to thyromental distance (RHTMD) improves the accuracy of predicting difficult laryngoscopy compared to TMD alone (sensitivity and specificity of 77% and 54%, respectively) (Krobbuaban et al. 2005).

The Wilson risk sum score (Wilson et al. 1988) takes five of the aforementioned factors into account and scores them between 0 and 2: the weight, the vertical head and neck movement, the jaw movement (prognathism), the receding mandible and buck teeth. In difficult laryngoscopy assessments, the true positive rate and false positive rate are influenced by changing the threshold values. In the original study, the authors proposed a threshold of 4, meaning a score greater than or equal to 4 indicates difficulty in intubation.

Prediction Methods applying AI are based on the listed parameters, with the general process being acquisition of facial features (or feature extraction) and output of the results using the acquired data. The whole process could be summarized as automatic face recognition. One of the most important stages in automatic face recognition is feature extraction. In the case of Espinoza-Cuadros et al., they posed the objective to have a specific compact and structured representation of craniofacial characteristics able to describe both inter- and intraclass variability for

OSA and non-OSA individuals. Three main types of facial features are included in automatic face recognition: holistic features, local features, and features derived by statistical models. They took the work from Lee et al. (2009a, b) as a reference, so local features are used. However, their major differences compared to the research in Lee et al. (2009a, b) are the use of supervised automatic image processing and the definition of more robust craniofacial measurements adapted to our less controlled photography capture process.

Identification of a set of relevant landmarks on images of subjects is the first critical step for extracting local facial features. Manual annotation of all images can be tedious and is prone to errors due to subjectivity even if done by skilled personnel. For this, there is a widely used automatic landmarking method first proposed by Cootes et al. in 2001 based on the Active Appearance Model (AAM) (Cootes et al. 2001; Teijeiro-Mosquera et al. 2010). The AAM is based on a priori knowledge of landmark locations, combined with a statistical model representing the shape and texture variation of the face (object), and uses a gradient-corrected fitting algorithm. They used a grid of 52 landmarks taken from general face recognition systems and a set of 24 landmarks including specific markers in the neck region in the AAM of frontal and profile photographs.

1.2 Speech Features Analysis in Difficult Airway Prediction

In addition to describing the compliance, shape, and dimensions of the upper airway, human speech also contains many characteristics of those structures. A narrow palate, a large tongue, a receding chin, and a limited opening of the mouth are all anatomical landmarks associated with difficult intubation, and these structural alterations may also affect pronunciation, making speech an excellent candidate for assessing difficult airways. Recent years have seen rapid advancements in speech technology. Since it is nonintrusive and provides objective data rapidly, it is becoming increasingly popular in various fields of medicine, including obstructive sleep apnea (OSA), depression, Parkinson's, and COVID-19. Yet, there is a scarcity of studies examining whether speech can lead to an accurate prediction of an airway obstruction. Earlier studies reported that speech may serve as an important diagnostic tool for difficult airways by de Carvalho et al. (2019a, b). Although the above studies did not use AI technology, speech recordings, and speech features were not comprehensive.

The author hypothesizes that the raw speech features and speaker recognition features extracted from syllables and sentences, combined with AI techniques, could be used to predict difficult airway. AI techniques mentioned in the previous sentence include machine learning, support vector machine, etc., with the general process being training, testing, and validating the data set, and the data set contains speech features in this case.

A speaker recognition system represents the acoustic information in an utterance by a sequence of feature vectors corresponding to the short-term spectral envelope of the sounds embedded within the utterance. The Mel-Frequency Cepstrum Coefficients (MFCC) are used in this study since most auto-speaker recognition systems use their first-order derivative (Kinnunen and Li 2010; Bimbot et al. 2004).

Further, since utterances exhibit different lengths of MFCC feature vectors, they are generally transformed into fixed-length vectors x that represent all the relevant acoustic information in the utterance (total variability is the vector space used to represent all the variability in that utterance). As a result, we will also be able to use a fixed-length acoustic vector x as input to the estimator function f, simplifying estimation.

This transformation is commonly conducted using i-vectors. A weighted sum of Gaussian component densities, Gaussian Mixture Models (GMM), were developed to model the probability density function of sequences of feature vectors. An adaptation of a universal background model (GMM-UBM) trained on a large speaker population can be used to generate a GMM representing an utterance from a particular speaker (Reynolds et al. 2000). A supervector is simply the stacked pile of all means of the adapted GMM that has been generated from a GMM-UBM using the utterances of a given speaker. Speech utterances will then be represented by high-dimensional vectors x of sizes 10–120 k, as the proportion of Gaussian components in a GMM for speaker recognition is typically 512–2048, and MFCC acoustic vector dimensions range from 20 to 60.

In addition to the advantage of projecting GMM supervectors into a low-dimensional subspace, i-vectors allow the user to capture more speaker-specific variability than supervectors do.

Both supervectors and i-vectors have successfully been used to recognize speakers (Dehak et al. 2011a), recognize languages (Dehak et al. 2011b), estimate speaker age (Bahari et al. 2014), estimate speaker height (Poorjam et al. 2014), and recognize accents (Bahari et al. 2013). Since speech contains significant sources of interfering intraspeaker variability (speaker weight, height, etc.), we believe the success of i-vectors in challenging tasks is a reasonable guarantee for their use in estimating the Apnea-Hypopnea Index. Due to the same microphone and four sentences read by all speakers, both channel and phonetic variations are minimized, so i-vectors can capture characteristics of sounds more affected by OSA, since the microphone was used for all recordings. In addition to discussing this topic in Espinoza-Cuadros et al. (2016), there is also a comparison of the use of i-vectors and supervectors when predicting the AHI.

2 AI and Intraoperative Airway Maintenance

2.1 Intraoperative Monitoring

Anesthesia monitoring and prediction AI is increasingly used in clinical anesthesia, and researchers have used algorithms to mine information from patient perioperative data, process and analyze multidimensional data, and develop predictive models to dynamically predict the occurrence of perioperative adverse events in order to improve patient perioperative safety.

Perioperative hypotension is associated with major cardiovascular adverse events as well as acute kidney injury (Hallqvist et al. 2018), and early prediction and early intervention of hypotension is a hot topic in current clinical research. Hatib et al. (2018) developed an AI algorithm for predicting hypotension based on arterial waveforms, and after validation, it was testified that using a large dataset of high-fidelity arterial waveforms, a machine learning model can be trained to predict arterial hypotension events in a surgical patient's physiologic dataset up to 15 minutes in advance.

The algorithm is also known as an early warning system. In view of the passive and lagging nature of this system for predicting hypotension, Wijnberge et al. (2020) proposed a new prediction model to assist physicians in proactively predicting the occurrence and cause of hypotension, which combines an early warning system with circulatory therapy guidelines, allowing anesthesiologists to quickly obtain potential causes of hypotension based on the parameters suggested by the computer system and corresponding to the flow chart. By intervening 15 min in advance of the etiology, the incidence of perioperative hypotension is effectively reduced and circulatory fluctuations during anesthesia are reduced.

The depth of anesthesia is associated with morbidity and mortality, postoperative adverse events and related organ damage, and maintaining the appropriate depth of anesthesia during the perioperative period is of great significance for clinical anesthesia. The current monitoring of perioperative depth of anesthesia is mainly based on the BIS, and maintaining the BIS at 40–60 can avoid intraoperative knowledge and deep anesthesia, but the BIS has a lag and is easily disturbed by the electric knife, which makes the monitoring effect vulnerable. The current research focuses on exploring methods to monitor the depth of perioperative anesthesia based on the patient's original EEG. Due to the complexity of EEG changes in different anesthesia states, it is difficult to effectively assess the depth of anesthesia by extracting a single feature. Extracted four effective parameters (entropy, EEG edge frequency, β-ratio, and relative synchronization of fast and slow waves) from EEG with the help of an artificial neural network, and used these four parameters as the input layer of the neural network and BIS as the output layer of the neural network to analyze the functional state of the brain, which can effectively distinguish the awake state from the anesthesia state of the patient; Gu et al. (2019) used wavelet transform method to analyze EEG and extract features. To further improve the accuracy of monitoring, Saadeh et al. (2019) used a machine learning classification processor to analyze the EEG and classified patients into four states: deep sedation, moderate sedation, light sedation, and awake, with an accuracy of 92.2% and a maximum lag time of 1 s. This method ensures that patients are appropriately anesthetized intraoperatively. This ensured the appropriate depth of anesthesia for the patient during surgery.

Researchers have also used AI to make other predictions, such as using neural networks to predict the recovery of muscle relaxation (Santanen et al. 2003); identifying patients with difficult tracheal intubation based on facial images (Cuendet et al. 2016b); and identifying patients with transfusion-related acute lung injury preoperatively (Murphree et al. 2015). intraoperative safety.

2.2 Drug Administration

2.2.1 Closed-Loop Target Controlled Injection

Total intravenous anesthesia (TIVA) has become readily accepted due to rapid-acting and stable anesthetics like propofol and remifentanil, which allow for rapid recovery. The use of target controlled infusion (TCI) has further improved TIVA, making it more compatible with the pharmacokinetics and pharmacodynamics of these drugs. TCI's pharmacokinetic model may not work in all patients because of individual differences. Propofol has been infusion controlled since the 1980s for this reason. Recently, many new closed-loop systems have been developed as a result of the development of computer technology and EEG monitoring technology. Infusions controlled by closed loops can avoid the limitations of TCI by compensating for individual differences, which allows anesthetics to be used rationally. Anesthesiologists may also be able to reduce their workload with closed-loop controlled infusions.

Electrocortical activity is altered by anesthetics in a dose-dependent manner. Several comparative studies have involved the infusion of propofol, and the bispectral index (BIS) has been widely used to monitor anesthesia depth and to regulate anesthetic administration during general anesthesia.

In clinical work, anesthesiologists need to adjust the dosage of drugs in real time according to the condition of patient and surgery, such as the stability of the patient's vital signs stable. In order to keep patients in a suitable state of sedation, analgesia, and neuromuscular relaxation are administered. Considering the characteristics of anesthesiologists' work that the infusion of various drugs should be closely regulated, researchers have developed an automated infusion system, which can automatically maintain the suitable state of anesthesia of patients. The system is called closed-loop target-controlled infusion system, referred to as a closed-loop system. The system consists of four components: (1) anesthesia effect parameters, which measure the degree of drug efficacy, such as BIS; (2) parameter set points, where the anesthesiologist pre-sets the control range of effect parameters; (3) a controller, where the computer processes the parameters through an algorithm and issues command to the actuator; and (4) an actuator, which is the drug infusion pump. The anesthesiologist can press the "pause" or "stop" button at any time during the working time of the system to stop it and control the anesthesia manually, so as to prevent unexpected events caused by loopholes and ensure patient safety.

The first attempt to use a closed-loop system happened in 1950 when Mayo et al. (1950) used EEG analysis to automate the management of thiopental sodium sedation. BIS automated control of propofol infusion, maintaining a BIS of 40–60 to ensure appropriate depth of sedation for the patient (Liu et al. 2012). As single-loop closed-loop systems become mature, more intelligent multi-loop closed-loop systems are developed to support the administration of anesthesia. For example, Liu et al. (2011) used BIS to control the infusion of remifentanil and propofol, and developed a dual-loop closed-loop system in which the target BIS value was set at 40–60, and only the infusion rate of remifentanil was adjusted when the BIS difference (actual BIS value and target BIS value) was 2–3 (if the infusion rate of remifentanil was changed for three consecutive times, the infusion rate of propofol was changed simultaneously); when the BIS difference was >4, the infusion rate of propofol and remifentanil would be changed, and the automated control of sedation and analgesia was successfully completed. To meet more anesthetic needs, Hemmerling et al. (2013a) developed the world's first fully automated closed-loop anesthesia infusion system, McSleepy, which uses BIS, Analgoscore, and four cascade stimuli as sedation, analgesia, and muscle relaxation parameters, respectively. The system has successfully automated the management of induction and maintenance of anesthesia in non-cardiac surgery by controlling the infusion of propofol, remifentanil, and rocuronium, respectively. Later, it was testified that the closed-loop system can be used not only for non-cardiac surgery, but also for cardiac surgery, pediatric anesthesia, and telemedicine with continuous optimization of the system (Biswas et al. 2013; Hemmerling et al. 2013b), expanding the application scenarios of the closed-loop system in the field of anesthesia. Studies have shown that compared with manual control, closed-loop systems have faster postoperative awakening, shorter extubation time, smoother anesthesia, and also reduced the occurrence of postoperative cognitive dysfunction in elderly patients (Besch et al. 2018).

In recent years, the value of closed-loop systems has not just been limited to anesthesia sedation, analgesia, and muscle relaxation, researchers have also developed closed-loop systems for perioperative fluid infusion and vasoactive drug administration. A closed-loop fluid infusion system is a closed-loop system that simulates the principles of goal-directed fluid infusion and automates the management of perioperative fluid infusion based on variables such as urine volume, blood pressure, heart rate, volume per beat, variability per beat, and pulse pressure variability (Rinehart et al. 2012). Variability, and automated control of remifentanil, propofol, crystalloid, and colloid infusions, promoting the diversification of closed-loop systems. The closed-loop system can also automatically control the infusion of vasoconstrictor (Joosten et al. 2019) or vasodilator (Mackenzie et al. 1993) according to the feedback of blood pressure and heart rate to maintain the target blood pressure. Yet due to the high development cost, imperfect safety assessment and the difficulty of clinical supervision, there are relatively few closed-loop systems developed on vasoactive drugs, and it is believed that in the future, with the development of engineering technology, closed-loop systems can combine more clinical indicators, truly simulate anesthesiologists and automate the perioperative anesthesia process.

2.2.2 Real-Time Control of Drug Administration

In recent times, many control engineers have been working toward developing a closed-loop control strategy for drug administration and scheduling to improve work efficiency, even in the presence of perturbations or uncertainties. Such techniques included PID, I-PD controllers, FLCs, PIDs with two degrees of freedom, fuzzy back-stepping controls with adaptive learning, adaptive control, closed-loop optimal controls, interval type-2 FLCs, MPCs, reinforcement learning controls, sliding mode controls (SMCs), super-twisting SMCs, and internal model controls (Bojkov et al. 1993; Algoul et al. 2011; El-Garawany et al. 2017; Khadraoui et al. 2016; Nasiri and Kalat 2018; Padmanabhan et al. 2017a,b; Sharifi and Moradi 2019; Ramkumar and Naidu 2007; Mahmoodian et al. 2015; Florian Jr et al. 2008; Sharifi et al. 2017; Dey et al. 2018; Kovács et al. 2014). In order to apply them on patients, clinical trials are the primary requirement for testing a new drug. It is important to note that protocols for determining the optimal dose of medication depend on a number of factors, including sex, weight, age, and body surface area. Pharmacokinetic changes arising from different patients are not taken into account by these factors (Karnik 2017). As part of chemotherapy treatment, a significant issue concerns the drug dose and time of administration. It is possible to lose efficacy (under-dosing) or cause toxicity (over-dosing) if the administered chemotherapeutic drug is nonconforming (Mage et al. 2017). To provide effective and reliable treatment for patients, a narrow and clear range of drugs must be administered. In 2017, Rokhforoz et al. developed a robust approach for the simultaneous control of cells such as immune cells, tumors, and normal cells by using an extended Kalman filter observer (Rokhforoz et al. 2017). During treatment sessions, the enhanced drug toxicity level is not taken into account when assessing the controller's stability. An in-depth analysis of currently available computational models for drug transport in tumors and other drug delivery methods, including nanoparticle-based and convection-enhanced methods, was published by Zhan et al. in 2018 (Zhan et al. 2018). The Lyapunov theory and Barbalat lemma are used to analyze the stability of closed-loop drug delivery (Khalili and Vatankhah 2019). In a study published in the *Journal of Applied Mathematics*, Panjwani et al. investigated the optimal scheduling of chemotherapy drugs using a PID control scheme with two degrees of freedom (Shindi et al. 2020). FLC can use expert knowledge to develop automated drug delivery systems. However, clinical trials are not included in any of these simulation studies and models. Clinical trials are needed to confirm the effectiveness of chemotherapeutic agents, taking into account hindering factors, interfering factors, individual pharmacokinetics, and pharmacodynamics (Pandey et al. 2018; Panjani et al. 2019; Karar and El-Brawany 2011; Yu et al. 2018).

Personalized devices have been revolutionized with MEMS technology, which is mentioned as a potential treatment for cancer. MEMS devices composed of polydimethylsiloxane were presented by Song et al. containing doxorubicin, which significantly inhibited pancreatic cancer cell growth (Song et al. 2013). Using intuitionistic fuzzy sets and optimization techniques, Karar et al. developed invasive weed optimization, a closed-loop FLC approach to control intravenous drug administration. Controlling the drug concentration using this method is optimal and adaptive. Researchers will use progressive patient models with drug side effects such as autoimmune reactions and cellular damage in the future. The ultimate goal of this work is to conduct real-time preclinical studies in animals using the developed controller.

It was proposed by Mage et al. in 2017 that chemotherapeutic agents could be administered in a real-time closed-loop system. In live rats and rabbits, they used an aptamer-based biosensor to demonstrate stable and prolonged closed-loop control of doxorubicin (Mage et al. 2017). Human clinical trials with chemotherapeutic agents can be conducted with real-time controlled drug delivery. This study, however, used a simple PID controller, which measured in vivo concentration output and compared it to a reference set point for calculating the rate of drug infusion. Control algorithms can be improved to achieve faster control of drug administration, according to the research. It may be better to use advanced control approaches such as model predictive control to restrict chemotherapeutic agents in real time, since they account for nonlinearities and self-adaptation based on patient-to-patient pharmacokinetic changes without requiring manual adjustments. A closed-loop control system for the treatment of cancer could also be provided by AI-based techniques.

3 Clinical Decision Support System

With the increasing popularity of AIMS, researchers have used machine learning to comprehensively analyze the comprehensive database of patient anesthesia and develop a hardware system that provides real-time decision aids for anesthesiologists to reduce physician errors, which is called Clinical Decision Support System (CDSS). The system mainly collects data from AIMS, categorizes the data into usable data by transformation, filtering, and missing fill, and the decision.

Anesthesia records are a major component of clinical anesthesia, and patient perioperative data can provide a reference for subsequent anesthesia management and case management. The current AIMS in major hospitals can collect data from sources such as monitors, hospital information systems, ventilators, and anesthesia workstations in real time, and anesthesiologists record the patient's fluid balance status, surgery, medication records, and special events in real time based on intraoperative anesthesia management, making the anesthesia record a comprehensive database of real-time information about the patient during surgery.

The decision processor applies algorithms to the data and determines whether to notify or alert (e.g., pop-up messages or flashing buttons) on the AIMS according to the decision rules that have been set. In the early days, CDSS was mainly used for routine workflow reminders, such as prompting physicians to give intraoperative antibiotics, beta-blockers, optimize ventilator parameters, avoid wasting anesthetic drugs, and check anesthesia bills (Freundlich and Ehrenfeld 2017). Ehrenfeld et al. developed a CDSS for intraoperative glucose monitoring, which uses an autoregressive algorithm to automatically identify potential diabetic patients using mathematical modeling based on patient demographics, disease history, type of anesthesia, surgical characteristics, insulin levels, and glucose levels (Ehrenfeld et al. 2017). The CDSS can also be used to identify the target population based on patient information from AIMS, such as brain injury traumatic pediatric patients undergoing neurosurgery, and remind anesthesiologists of the key points of anesthesia to focus on intraoperative process according to the set algorithm rules, reducing the incidence of intraoperative adverse events (Kiatchai et al. 2017). However, the reminder interface of the early CDSS is monotonous and sometimes difficult to attract anesthesiologists' attention. The new CDSS integrates the patient's circulatory indexes, respiratory parameters, fluid balance, laboratory test results, and alarm reminders in a single reminder interface with different colored organ dynamic diagrams, which comprehensively and vividly reflects the patients' intraoperative situation and improves the anesthesiologists' perioperative management efficiency (Kheterpal et al. 2018).

Most of the current CDSS are reactive support systems, and researchers developing new systems can collect data from monitors directly while processing large amounts of data streams with the help of 5G networks to develop CDSS with real-time prediction, but such predictive CDSS are still in the research stage.

As part of AI-enabled CDSS, intelligent components are included, representing a paradigm shift compared with traditional CDSS (Sim et al. 2001; Haynes and Wilczynski 2010; Grout et al. 2018; Jia et al. 2020; Daniel et al. 2019; Salem et al. 2015). Using sophisticated algorithms, they transform raw medical data, documents, and expert practice into a set of tools that assist clinicians. In this way, users can find suitable solutions to their medical problems and make clinical decisions using machine learning, knowledge graphs, natural language processing, and computer vision (Aljaaf et al. 2015). In addition to improving clinician performance, quality of health care, and patient safety, AI-enabled CDSS can also save costs for healthcare payers (Richard et al. 2020).

The use of AI-enabled CDSS in diagnostics is significant, especially in the diagnosis of rare diseases, the detection and prediction of sepsis, fracture detection, and the treatment of cancers (Faviez et al. 2020; Wulff et al. 2019; Langerhuizen et al. 2019; Yassin et al. 2018; Ferrante di Ruffano et al. 2018). The use of AI-assisted CDSS has also been documented for the management of health care and medication therapy (Roumeliotis et al. 2019; Rawson et al. 2017; Oluoch et al. 2012; Carter et al. 2019).

A CDSS enabled by AI will be able to learn from actual use and experience (training) and improve its performance (adaptation) (Tang 2019). AI can handle large amounts of text classification, information retrieval, and information extraction from hospital electronic health records by using techniques such as knowledge graphs and natural language processing. The use of AI can facilitate clinicians' ability to make more comprehensive and personalized decisions based on structured data through techniques such as machine learning. Another benefit is that the functionality and utility of CDSS combined with AI techniques outperform those of traditional systems, and through intelligent behavior patterns and the ability to learn new clinical knowledge, the system improves and supports the decision-making process (Aljaaf et al. 2015).

References

Ahn H-I, Picard RW. Measuring affective-cognitive experience and predicting market success. IEEE trans. Affective computing. 2014;

Algoul S, Alam MS, Hossain MA, Majumder MA. Multiobjective optimal chemotherapy control model for cancer treatment. Med Biol Eng Comput. 2011;49:51–65.

Aljaaf A, Al-Jumeily D, Hussain A, Fergus P, Al-Jumaily M, Abdel-Aziz K. Toward an optimal use of artificial intelligence techniques within a clinical decision support system. Science and information conference., London, UK. 2015.

Aziz MF, et al. Routine clinical practice effectiveness of the glidescope in difficult airway management: an analysis of 2,004 glidescope intubations, complications, and failures from two institutions. Anesthesiology. 2011;114(1):34–41.

Bahari MH, Saeidi R, Van Hamme H, Van Leeuwen D. Accent recognition using i-vector, Gaussian mean supervector and gaussian posterior probability supervector for spontaneous telephone speech. In: Proceedings of the 38th IEEE international conference on acoustics, speech, and signal processing (ICASSP'13). Vancouver, Canada: IEEE; 2013. p. 7344–8.

Bahari MH, McLaren M, van Hamme H, van Leeuwen DA. Speaker age estimation using i-vectors. Eng Appl Artif Intell. 2014;34:99–108.

Baker PA, Depuydt A, Thompson JMD. Thyromental distance measurement – fingers don't rule. Anaesthesia. 2009;64(8):878–82.

Baynam G, et al. Intersections of epigenetics, twinning and developmental asymmetries: insights into monogenic and complex diseases and a role for 3d facial analysis. Twin Res Hum Genet. 2011;14(4):305–15.

Besch G, Vettoretti L, Claveau M, et al. Early postoperative cognitive dysfunction after closed-loop versus manual target controlled-infusion of propofol and remifentanil in patients undergoing elective major non-cardiac surgery: protocol of the randomized controlled single-blind POCD-ELA trial. Medicine (Baltimore). 2018;97(40):e12558.

Bimbot F, Bonastre J-F, Fredouille C, et al. A tutorial on textindependent speaker verification. EURASIP J Appl Signal Process. 2004;2004(4) 101962:430–51.

Biswas I, Mathew PJ, Singh RS, et al. Evaluation of closed-loop anesthesia delivery for propofol anesthesia in pediatric cardiac surgery. Paediatr Anaesth. 2013;23(12):1145–52.

Bojkov B, Hansel R, Luus R. Application of direct search optimization to optimal control problems. Hung J Ind Chem. 1993;21(3):177–85.

Carter J, Sandall J, Shennan AH, Tribe RM. Mobile phone apps for clinical decision support in pregnancy: a scoping review. BMC Med Inform Decis Mak. 2019;19(1):219. https://doi.org/10.1186/s12911-019-0954-1. https://bmcmedinformdecismak.biomedcentral.com/articles/10.1186/s12911-019-0954-1.

Cattano D, et al. Risk factors assessment of the difficult airway: an italian survey of 1956 patients. Anesth Analg. 2004;99(6):1774–9.

Cevikalp H, Triggs B, Franc V. Face and landmark detection by using cascade of classifiers. In: 10nth IEEE int. conf. automat. Face and Gesture Recognition; 2013.

Claes P, et al. Dysmorphometrics: the modelling of morphological abnormalities. Theor Biol Med Model. 2012;9(1):5.

Cook TM, Macdougall-Davis SR. Complications and failure of airway management. Br J Anaesth. 2012;109:i68–85.

Cootes TF, Edwards GJ, Taylor CJ. Active appearance models. IEEE Trans Pattern Anal Mach Intell. 2001;23(6):681–5.

Cuendet GL, et al. Facial image analysis for fully automatic prediction of difficult endotracheal intubation. IEEE Trans Biomed Eng. 2016a;63(2):328–39. https://doi.org/10.1109/TBME.2015.2457032.

Cuendet GL, Schoettker P, Yüce A, et al. Facial image analysis for fully automatic prediction of difficult endotracheal intubation. IEEE Trans Biomed Eng. 2016b;63(2):328–39.

Daniel G, Silcox C, Sharma I, Wright M. Current state and near-term priorities for ai-enabled diagnostic support software in health care. Duke Margolis Center for Health Policy; 2019.

de Carvalho CC, da Silva DM, de Carvalho Junior AD, et al. Pre-operative voice evaluation as a hypothetical predictor of difficult laryngoscopy. Anaesthesia. 2019a;74:1147–52.

de Carvalho CC, da Silva DM, de Carvalho AD, FJF N Jr, de Orange FA. Evaluation of the association between voice formants and difficult facemask ventilation. Eur J Anaesthesiol. 2019b;36:972–3.

Dehak N, Kenny PJ, Dehak R, Dumouchel P, Ouellet P. Front-end factor analysis for speaker verification. IEEE Trans Audio Speech Lang Process. 2011a;19(4):788–98.

Dehak N, Torres-Carrasquillo PA, Reynolds D, Dehak R. Language recognition via Ivectors and dimensionality reduction. In: Proceedings of the 12th annual conference of the international speech communication association (INTERSPEECH'11). Florence, Italy; 2011b. p. 857–60.

Dey BS, Bera MK, Roy BK. Super twisting sliding mode control of cancer chemotherapy: 15th international workshop on variable structure systems (VSS). Graz, Austria: Graz University of Technology; 2018. p. 343–34.

Dong Y, et al. Driver inattention monitoring system for intelligent vehicles: a review. In: Proc. IEEE intelligent vehicles symp; 2009. p. 875–80.

Eberhart LHJ, et al. The reliability and validity of the upper lip bite test compared with the mallampati classification to predict difficult laryngoscopy: an external prospective evaluation. Anesth Analg. 2005;101(1):284–9.

Ehrenfeld JM, Wanderer JP, Terekhov M, et al. A perioperative systems design to improve intraoperative glucose monitoring is associated with a reduction in surgical site infections in a diabetic patient population. Anesthesiology. 2017;126(3):431–40.

El-Garawany AH, Karar ME, El-Brawany MA. Embedded drug delivery controller for cancer chemotherapy under treatment constraints. In: Intl conf on advanced control circuits systems (ACCS) systems & 2017 intl conf on new Paradigms in Electronics & Information Technology (PEIT), 2017. Egypt: Alexandria; 2017.

Espinoza-Cuadros F, Fern'andez-Pozo R, Toledano DT, Alc'azar-Ram'ırez JD, L'opez-Gonzalo E, Hern'andez- G'omez L. Reviewing the connection between speech and obstructive sleep apnea. Biomed Eng Online. 2016;15:20. In press.

Faviez C, Chen X, Garcelon N, Neuraz A, Knebelmann B, Salomon R, Lyonnet S, Saunier S, Burgun A. Diagnosis support systems for rare diseases: a scoping review. Orphanet J Rare Dis. 2020;15(1):94. https://doi.org/10.1186/s13023-020-01374-z.

Ferrante di Ruffano L, Takwoingi Y, Dinnes J, Chuchu N, Bayliss SE, Davenport C, Matin RN, Godfrey K, O'Sullivan C, Gulati A, Chan SA, Durack A, O'Connell S, Gardiner MD, Bamber J, Deeks JJ, Williams HC. Cochrane skin cancer diagnostic test accuracy group computer-assisted diagnosis techniques (dermoscopy and spectroscopy-based) for diagnosing skin cancer in adults. Cochrane Database Syst Rev. 2018;12:CD013186. https://doi.org/10.1002/14651858.CD013186.

Florian JA Jr, Eiseman JL, Parker RS. Nonlinear model predictive control for dosing daily anticancer agents using a novel saturating-rate cell-cycle model. Comput Biol Med. 2008;38:339–47.

Freundlich RE, Ehrenfeld JM. Anesthesia information management: clinical decision support. Curr Opin Anaesthesiol. 2017;30(6):705–9.

Gao H, Yuce A, Thiran J-P. Detecting emotional stress from facial expressions for driving safety. In: Proc. int. conf. on image process; 2014.

Grout RW, Cheng ER, Carroll AE, Bauer NS, Downs SM. A six-year repeated evaluation of computerized clinical decision support system user acceptability. Int J Med Inform. 2018;112:74–81. https://doi.org/10.1016/j.ijmedinf.2018.01.011.

Gu Y, Liang Z, Hagihira S. Use of multiple EEG features and artificial neural network to monitor the depth of anesthesia. Sensors (Basel). 2019;19(11):2499.

Hallqvist L, Granath F, Huldt E, et al. Intraoperative hypotension is associated with acute kidney injury in noncardiac surgery: an observational study. Eur J Anaesthesiol. 2018;35(4):273–9.

Hatib F, Jian Z, Buddi S, et al. Machine-learning algorithm to predict hypotension based on high-fidelity arterial pressure waveform analysis. Anesthesiology. 2018;129(4):663–74.

Hayasaka T, Kawano K, Kurihara K, Suzuki H, Nakane M, Kawamae K. Creation of an artificial intelligence model for intubation difficulty classification by deep learning (convolutional neural network) using face images: an observational study. J Intensive Care. 2021;9(1):38.

Haynes RB, Wilczynski NL. Computerized clinical decision support system (CCDSS) systematic review team effects of computerized clinical decision support systems on practitioner performance and patient outcomes: methods of a decision-maker-researcher partnership systematic review. Implement Sci. 2010;5:12. https://doi.org/10.1186/1748-5908-5-12.

Heard AMB, Green RJ, Eakins P. The formulation and introduction of a 'can't intubate, can't ventilate' algorithm into clinical practice. Anaesthesia. 2009;64(6):601–8.

Hemmerling TM, Arbeid E, Wehbe M, et al. Evaluation of a novel closed-loop total intravenous anaesthesia drug delivery system: a randomized controlled trial. Br J Anaesth. 2013a;110(6):1031–9.

Hemmerling TM, Arbeid E, Wehbe M, et al. Transcontinental anaesthesia: a pilot study. Br J Anaesth. 2013b;110(5):758–63.

Hove LD, et al. Analysis of deaths related to anesthesia in the period 1996–2004 from closed claims registered by the Danish patient insurance association. Anesthesiology. 2007;106(4):675–80.

Jia P, Jia P, Chen J, Zhao P, Zhang M. The effects of clinical decision support systems on insulin use: a systematic review. J Eval Clin Pract. 2020;26(4):1292–301. https://doi.org/10.1111/jep.13291.

Joosten A, Delaporte A, Alexander B, et al. Automated titration of vasopressor infusion using a closed-loop controller: in vivo feasibility study using a swine model. Anesthesiology. 2019;130(3):394–403.

Karar ME, El-Brawany MA. Automated cardiac drug infusion system using adaptive fuzzy neural networks controller. Biomed Eng Comput Biol. 2011;3:BECB-S6495.

Karnik R. Drug delivery: closed-loop dynamic dosing. Nat Biomed Eng. 2017;1(5):0073.

Khadraoui S, Harrou F, Nounou HN, Nounou MN, Datta A, Bhattacharya SP. A measurement-based control design approach for efficient cancer chemotherapy. Inf Sci. 2016;333:108–25.

Khalili P, Vatankhah R. Derivation of an optimal trajectory and nonlinear adaptive controller design for drug delivery in cancerous tumor chemotherapy. Comput Biol Med. 2019;109:195–206.

Khan ZH, Kashfi A, Ebrahimkhani E. A comparison of the upper lip bite test (a simple new technique) with modified mallampati classification in predicting difficulty in endotracheal intubation: a prospective blinded study. Anesth Analg. 2003;96(2):595–9.

Khan ZH, et al. The diagnostic value of the upper lip bite test combined with sternomental distance, thyromental distance, and interincisor distance for prediction of easy laryngoscopy and intubation: a prospective study. Anesth Analg. 2009;109(3):822–4.

Kheterpal S, Shanks A, Tremper KK. Impact of a novel multiparameter decision support system on intraoperative processes of care and postoperative outcomes. Anesthesiology. 2018;128(2):272–82.

Kiatchai T, Colletti AA, Lyons VH, et al. Development and feasibility of a real-time clinical decision support system for traumatic brain injury anesthesia care. Appl Clin Inform. 2017;8(1):80–96.

Kinnunen T, Li H. An overview of text-independent speaker recognition: from features to supervectors. Speech Comm. 2010;52(1):12–40.

Kovács L, Szeles A, Sápi J, Drexler DA, Rudas I, Harmati I, Sápi Z. Model-based angiogenic inhibition of tumor growth using modern robust control method. Comput Meth Prog Biomed. 2014;114(3):98–110.

Krobbuaban B, et al. The predictive value of the height ratio and thyromental distance: four predictive tests for difficult laryngoscopy. Anesth Analg. 2005;101(5):1542–5.

Langerhuizen DWG, Janssen SJ, Mallee WH, van den Bekerom MPJ, Ring D, Kerkhoffs GMMJ, Jaarsma RL, Doornberg JN. What are the applications and limitations of artificial intelligence for fracture detection and classification in orthopaedic trauma imaging? A systematic review. Clin Orthop Relat Res. 2019;477(11):2482–91. https://doi.org/10.1097/CORR.0000000000000848.

Lee A, et al. A systematic review (meta-analysis) of the accuracy of the mallampati tests to predict the difficult airway. Anesth Analg. 2006;102(6):1867–78.

Lee RWW, Chan ASL, Grunstein RR, Cistulli PA. Craniofacial phenotyping in obstructive sleep apnea-a novel quantitative photographic approach. Sleep. 2009a;32(1):37–45.

Lee RWW, Petocz P, Prvan T, Chan ASL, Grunstein RR, Cistulli PA. Prediction of obstructive sleep apnea with craniofacial photographic analysis. Sleep. 2009b;32(1):46–52.

Liu N, Chazot T, Hamada S, et al. Closed-loop coadministration of propofol and remifentanil guided by bispectral index: a randomized multicenter study. Anesth Analg. 2011;112(3):546–57.

Liu N, Le Guen M, Benabbes-Lambert F, et al. Feasibility of closed-loop titration of propofol and remifentanil guided by the spectral M-entropy monitor. Anesthesiology. 2012;116(2):286–95.

Lundstrøm LH, et al. Poor prognostic value of the modified mallampati score: a meta-analysis involving 177 088 patients. Br J Anaesth. 2011;107(5):659–67.

Mackenzie AF, Colvin JR, Kenny GN, et al. Closed loop control of arterial hypertension following intracranial surgery using sodium nitroprusside. A comparison of intra-operative halothane or isoflurane. Anaesthesia. 1993;48(3):202–4.

Mage PL, Ferguson BS, Maliniak D, Ploense KL, Kippin TE, Soh HT. Closed-loop control of circulating drug levels in live animals. Nat Biomed Eng. 2017;1:0070.

Mahmoodian H, Salem S, Shojaei K, Adaptively adjusted footprint of uncertainty in interval type-2 fuzzy controller for cancer drug delivery. In IEEE International Symposium on Robotics and Intelligent Sensors. Procedia Comput Sci 2015; 2015(76): 360–367.

Mayo CW, Bickford RG, Faulconer A Jr. Electroencephalographically controlled anesthesia in abdominal surgery. J Am Med Assoc. 1950;144(13):1081–3.

Metzner J, et al. Closed claims' analysis. Best Pract Res Clin Anaesthesiol. 2011;25(2):263–76.

Murphree D, Ngufor C, Upadhyaya S, et al. Ensemble learning approaches to predicting complications of blood transfusion. Annu Int Conf IEEE Eng Med Biol Soc. 2015;2015:7222–5.

Nasiri H, Kalat AA. Adaptive fuzzy back-stepping control of drug dosage regimen in cancer treatment. Biomed Signal Process Control. 2018;42:267–76.

Oluoch T, Santas X, Kwaro D, Were M, Biondich P, Bailey C, Abu-Hanna A, de KN. The effect of electronic medical record-based clinical decision support on HIV care in resource-constrained settings: a systematic review. Int J Med Inform. 2012;81(10):e83–92. https://doi.org/10.1016/j.ijmedinf.2012.07.010.

Padmanabhan R, Meskin N, Haddad WM. Learning-based control of cancer chemotherapy treatment. IFAC PapersOnLine. 2017a;50(1):15127–32.

Padmanabhan R, Meskin N, Haddad WM. Reinforcement learning-based control of drug dosing for cancer chemotherapy treatment. Math Biosci. 2017b;293:11–20.

Pandey V, Pachauri N, Ran A, Rani V, Single V. Optimal ISAPID- based drug concentration control in cancer chemotherapy. In: Book chapter in advances in intelligent systems and computing; 2018. p. 165–71.

Panjani B, Mohan V, Rani A, Singh V. Optimal drug scheduling for cancer chemotherapy using two-degree of freedom fractional order PID scheme. J Intell Fuzzy Syst. 2019;36(3):2273–84.

Poorjam A, Bahari M, Vasilakakis V, Van-Hamme H. Height estimation from speech signals using i-vectors and least-squares support vector regression. In: Proceedings of the 37th international conference on telecommunications and signal processing (TSP '14); 2014. p. 1–5., Berlin, Germany.

Ramkumar B, Naidu DS. Closed-loop optimal control strategy for cancer chemotherapy. In: Proceedings of IMECE, 2007 ASME international mechanical engineering congress and exposition.; Seattle, Washington, USA; 2007.

Rawson TM, Moore LSP, Hernandez B, Charani E, Castro-Sanchez E, Herrero P, Hayhoe B, Hope W, Georgiou P, Holmes AH. A systematic review of clinical decision support systems for antimicrobial management: are we failing to investigate these interventions appropriately? Clin Microbiol Infect. 2017;23(8):524–32. https://doi.org/10.1016/j.cmi.2017.02.028. https://linkinghub.elsevier.com/retrieve/pii/S1198-743X(17)30125-8.

Reynolds DA, Quatieri TF, Dunn RB. Speaker verification using adapted Gaussian mixture models. Digit Signal Process. 2000;10(1):19–41.

Richard A, Mayag B, Talbot F, Tsoukias A, Meinard Y. What does it mean to provide decision support to a responsible and competent expert? Euro J Decis Process. 2020;8(3–4):205–36. https://doi.org/10.1007/s40070-020-00116-7.

Rinehart J, Chung E, Canales C, et al. Intraoperative stroke volume optimization using stroke volume, arterial pressure, and heart rate: closed-loop (earning intravenous resuscitator) versus anesthesiologists. J Cardiothorac Vasc Anest. 2012;26(5):933–9.

Ringeval F, et al. Prediction of asynchronous dimensional emotion ratings from audiovisual and physiological data. Pattern Recognition Lett. 2014;66:22–30.

Rokhforoz P, Jamshidi AA, Sarvestani NN. Adaptive robust control of cancer chemotherapy with extended Kalman filter observer. Inform Med Unlocked. 2017;8:1–7.

Roumeliotis N, Sniderman J, Adams-Webber T, Addo N, Anand V, Rochon P, Taddio A, Parshuram C. Effect of electronic prescribing strategies on medication error and harm in hospital: a systematic review and meta-analysis. J Gen Intern Med. 2019;34(10):2210–23. https://doi.org/10.1007/s11606-019-05236-8. http://europepmc.org/abstract/MED/31396810.

Saadeh W, Khan FH, Altaf MAB. Design and implementation of a machine learning based EEG processor for accurate estimation of depth of anesthesia. IEEE Trans Biomed Circuits Syst. 2019;13(4):658–69.

Salem H, Attiya G, El-Fishawy N. A survey of multi-agent based intelligent decision support system for medical classification problems. Int J Comput Appl. 2015;123(10):20–5. https://doi.org/10.5120/ijca2015905529.

Santanen OA, Svartling N, Haasio J, et al. Neural nets and prediction of the recovery rate from neuromuscular block. Eur J Anaesthesiol. 2003;20(2):87–92.

Serocki G, et al. Management of the predicted difficult airway: a comparison of conventional blade laryngoscopy with video-assisted blade laryngoscopy and the glidescope. Eur J Anaesthesiol. 2010;27(1):24–30.

Sharifi M, Moradi H. Nonlinear composite adaptive control of cancer chemotherapy with online identification of uncertain parameters. Biomed Signal Process Control. 2019;49:360–74.

Sharifi N, Ozgoli S, Ramezani A. Multiple model predictive control for optimal drug administration of mixed immunotherapy and chemotherapy of tumours. Comput Meth Prog Biomed. 2017;144:13–9.

Shindi O, Kanesan J, Kendall G, Ramanathan A. The combined effect of optimal control and swarm intelligence on optimization of cancer chemotherapy. Comput Methods Prog Biomed. 2020;189:105327.

Sim I, Gorman P, Greenes RA, Haynes RB, Kaplan B, Lehmann H, Tang PC. Clinical decision support systems for the practice of evidence-based medicine. J Am Med Inform Assoc. 2001;8(6):527–34.

Song P, Tng DJH, Hu R, Lin G, Meng E, Yong KT. An electrochemically actuated MEMS device for individualized drug delivery: an in vitro study. Adv Healthc Mater. 2013;2(8):1170–8.

Tang H. Proposed regulatory framework for modifications to artificial intelligence/machine learning (AI/ML)-based software as a medical device (SAMD) – discussion paper and request for feedback. US Food and Drug Administration; 2019.

Teijeiro-Mosquera L, Alba-Castro JL, Gonz'alez-Jim'enez D. Face recognition across pose with automatic estimation of pose parameters through AAM-based landmarking. In: Proceedings of the 20th international conference on pattern recognition (ICPR '10); 2010. p. 1339–42., Istanbul, Turkey.

Teoh WHL, et al. Comparison of three videolaryngoscopes: pentax airway scope, c-macTM, glidescope R vs the macintosh laryngoscope for tracheal intubation. Anaesthesia. 2010;65(11):1126–32.

Wijnberge M, Geerts BF, Hol L, et al. Effect of a machine learning-derived early warning system for intraoperative hypotension vs standard care on depth and duration of intraoperative hypotension during elective noncardiac surgery: the hype randomized clinical trial. JAMA. 2020;323(11):1052–60.

Wilson ME, et al. Predicting difficult intubation. Br J Anaesth. 1988;61(2):211–6.

Wulff A, Montag S, Marschollek M, Jack T. Clinical decision-support systems for detection of systemic inflammatory response syndrome, sepsis, and septic shock in critically ill patients: a systematic review. Methods Inf Med. 2019;58(S 02):e43–57. https://doi.org/10.1055/s-0039-1695717. http://www.thieme-connect.com/DOI/DOI?10.1055/s-0039-1695717.

Xiong X, De La Torre F. Supervised descent method and its applications to face alignment. In: Proc. IEEE Comput. Soc. Conf. on Comput. Vision and pattern recognition; 2013. p. 532–9.

Yassin NIR, Omran S, El Houby EMF, Allam H. Machine learning techniques for breast cancer computer aided diagnosis using different image modalities: a systematic review. Comput Methods Prog Biomed. 2018;156:25–45. https://doi.org/10.1016/j.cmpb.2017.12.012.

Yu YN, Doctor F, Fan SZ, Shieh JS. An adaptive monitoring scheme for automatic control of anaesthesia in dynamic surgical environments based on bispectral index and blood pressure. J Med Syst. 2018;42(5):95.

Zhan W, Alamer M, Xu XY. Computational modelling of drug delivery to solid tumour: understanding the interplay between chemotherapeutics and biologi-

cal system for optimized delivery systems. Adv Drug Deliv Rev. 2018;132(81):1–3.
Zhao Q, et al. Automated down syndrome detection using facial photographs. In: Proc. Annu. Int. conf. IEEE Eng. medicine and biology Soc.; 2013.
Zhu X, Ramanan D. Face detection, pose estimation, and landmark localization in the wild. In: Proc. IEEE Comput. Soc. Conf. on Comput. Vision and pattern recognition; 2012. p. 2879–86.

Artificial Intelligence in Prediction for Intraoperative Hypotension and Hypoxemia

Shuang Cao

There are attentive studies focusing on the direction of AI applications for adverse event monitoring. Generally, hazardous events can be broadly divided into two categories, those that can be quantified and those that cannot. For the quantifiable ones, such as hypotension and hypoxemia that we will explore in this chapter, they are expected to be predictable and interpretable; for the hard-to-quantify ones such as ataxic respiration and pain control that will be covered in other parts of this book, we want them to be quantifiable. To achieve the goal that we set for our management of hazardous events, we turned our direction toward AI technologies by combing the literature that may provide insights.

1 From Quantifiable to Predictable and Explainable Adverse Events

Take hypoxemia as an example, pulse oximetry can continuously detect SpO_2. Whereas, the indicator can only reflect real-time oxygen deficiency and cannot predict and prevent possible future oxygen deficiency. Previously, researchers have used machine learning to predict adverse events such as sepsis with adequate accuracy, but the problem is that the predictions are difficult to interpret. In other words, we are not sure why the adverse event occurred. The previous solution was to avoid complex but more accurate models and retreat to simpler interpretable models but at the cost of a decrease in accuracy. This reveals that accuracy and interpretation of the prediction are not available at the same time.

In 2018, Lundberg et al. built on recent advances in prediction interpretation methods for model uncertainty by developing a method that provides a theoretically sound explanation for model predictions that balances prediction accuracy and interpretability (Lundberg et al. 2018). This approach relies on the change when clinicians observe a feature (e.g., a patient's BMI) versus when clinicians do not observe that feature (e.g., not knowing the patient's BMI). The change in the model output prediction when a feature is observed indicates its importance to the prediction. This importance represents more of a correlation than a causality. However, by understanding these characteristics that are strongly correlated with risk prediction, clinicians can make preliminary interpretations in the context of clinical experience.

In achieving the prediction of hypoxemia, physicians can then adjust the parameter of inhaled oxygen content of the ventilator in advance to maintain blood oxygen concentration. Radhakrishnan et al. developed a system to

S. Cao (✉)
Department of Anesthesiology, Shanghai Ninth People's Hospital, Shanghai Jiao Tong University School of Medicine, Shanghai, China

M. Xia, H. Jiang (eds.), *Artificial Intelligence in Anesthesiology*,
https://doi.org/10.1007/978-981-99-5925-9_6

predict the FiO_2 required to maintain oxygen saturation, and the predicted output of this system was compared with the physician's decision and found the error to be less than 5% (Radhakrishnan et al. 2019). The same is true for hypotension, where a sphygmomanometer can measure blood pressure but cannot predict it. Kang et al. developed a machine learning model to predict anesthesia-induced hypotension that occurs during tracheal intubation to incision and found that the most important features affecting the accuracy of machine learning predictions were the patient's lowest SBP, lowest MAP, and mean SBP before tracheal intubation (Kang et al. 2020). In 2020, Cherifa et al. predicted acute hypotensive episodes 10 min in advance using the super learner algorithm (Cherifa et al. 2020).

2 Artificial Intelligence in Prediction for Intraoperative Hypotension

Intraoperative hypotension, defined as a mean arterial pressure (MAP) below 65 mmHg, is associated with an increased incidence of postoperative myocardial infarction and acute kidney injury, both of which are predictors of poor long-term patient prognosis. In the intensive care unit setting, hypotension is associated with an increased incidence of acute kidney injury. The risk of serious complications increases with the duration of hypotension, but it can begin to develop in as little as a few minutes. It is caused by anesthetics, pre-operative use of medication, existing comorbidities, pre-induction hypotension, or the surgery itself. Early warning of impending hypotension, even if the warning is given only 10–15 min in advance, can facilitate diagnostic and therapeutic measures to reduce the clinical impact.

Intraoperative arterial hypotension occurs frequently and is associated with postoperative morbidity and mortality. Hypotension in the early stage of anesthesia, known as post-induction hypotension (PIH), is associated with multiple causative mechanisms, such as the patient's age, pre-induction systolic blood pressure (SBP), and emergency surgery. Apart from these factors, comorbidities, medications used preoperatively, and anesthetic techniques, including the type and dose of anesthetic agent, can contribute to PIH. In light of these complex causes, predicting hypotension during induction of anesthesia has been challenging. Recognition of hypotensive events in a timely manner may be accomplished by machine learning algorithms, bringing early treatment and avoidance of adverse outcomes.

Kang et al. studied the feasibility of developing a machine learning model to predict PIH. If PIH could be accurately anticipated, anesthesiologists would be capable of proactively determine appropriate management strategies, so to avoid negative outcomes associated with hypotension. Over the years, modern anesthesia data have expanded to include high-resolution time-synchronized physiological and pharmacological data from multiple anesthesia devices. As a result, a wealth of anesthesia-related data to the traditional electronic health records; however, analyzing these data in real time to predict the occurrence of PIH in a busy operating room setting can be distracting to anesthesiologists. With this in mind, machine learning can be used as an alternative approach to assist anesthesiologists in using this data to predict PIH. Various machine learning models have been introduced to predict postoperative in-hospital mortality, hypotension, and PIH, whose predictive performance is equal to or outweighs traditional modeling (Kang et al. 2020).

Kang et al. developed Naïve Bayes, logistic regression, random forest, and artificial neural network (ANN) models for predicting late PIH. Naïve Bayes is a probabilistic classifier that applies the Bayesian theorem, which assumes independence between attributes. Logistic regression is a probabilistic model that uses the relationship between the dependent and independent variables as a specific function of the predictive model. Random forest randomly samples the training data to create a large number of decision trees and then collects the results of the decision trees to arrive at the final result by majority voting. The decision tree predicts the value of the target variable based on several input variables. Random forest has a high accuracy because it brings large amounts of these decision trees, learns them collectively, and comes up with a majority result. Convenient and rapid, it can deal with large data sets and many input variables. ANN simulates the information processing system of the human brain, involving complex neuronal connections and sophisticated computations. When various information is input, the ANN originates a new value through a predetermined functional process. Any estimated function can be approximated by a reasonably complex neural network with high prediction accuracy, which is the advantage of this algorithm. The authors performed iterative k-fold cross-validation to guarantee unbiased performance. Such a validation method is a statistical skill that measures the performance of the model on new data after dividing the data into k folds. A fold is tested as new data for the model built from the remaining k-1 folds, and the process is repeated while all folds are tested once. K-fold validation has random sample selection when forming a fold. When the samples are homogeneous, randomness will not lead to biased performance on a particular fold segmentation. Whereas, the performance of the algorithm may change when the samples are heterogeneous, according to which samples are split into which folds. The repeated k-fold validation complements this weakness by repeating the step of splitting the samples into folds. Biomedical data, especially our biosensor data, varies from patient to patient; thus the authors repeated the fourfold cross-validation 1000 times to produce stable performance.

Their evaluation result showed that machine learning can predict late PIH with a variable range; the random forest model achieved the best performance (AUC = 0.84) among the four methods tested. Selected features obtained through a feature selection method (20 and 23 features) performed better than using all 89 features. The three most important features affecting the prediction accuracy of machine learning (e.g., random forest) were the patient's lowest SBP, the lowest MBP, and the mean SBP before tracheal intubation. Among the patient features, the patient's age was an important factor in predicting advanced PIH (Kang et al. 2020).

In a narrative review, Van der Ven et al. described the Hypotension Prediction Index (HPI), one of the first machine learning (ML)-derived prediction algorithms for use in the operating room setting (Van der Ven et al. 2021). The HPI is a unitless number that ranges from 1 to 100, and as the number increases, the risk of an event occurring in the future increases. The potential value of the HPI in clinical use is to provide anesthesiologists with real-time information that allows them to proactively address impending hypotensive events. The overview discusses the development and validation process, advantages, limitations, and potential clinical utility of HPI. The HPI is a supervised ML algorithm that is trained to classify outputs to predict a desired or undesired event.

HPI performance was assessed in two retrospective trials and two clinical randomized controlled trials. One of these retrospective analyses validated HPI performance in 255 patients undergoing major surgery, with predictions close to the actual onset of hypotension within the first 5, 10, or 15 min before hypotension occurs, with AUCs of 0.93, 0.90, and 0.88, respectively (Davies et al. 2020). In another small retrospective study of 23 patients undergoing vascular or cardiac surgery, HPI performance was worse, with an AUC of 0.77 when predicting hypotension 5–7 min before its onset (Ranucci et al. 2019).

Moreover, a prospective study, an RCT of patients scheduled for hip arthroplasty, compared 25 patients receiving goal-directed hemodynamic therapy such as the administration of colloid and/or vascular compressors, with 24 patients treated with routine care. Time to hypotension was significantly reduced in the intervention group (0% vs 6% of total anesthesia time, $P < 0.001$). According to the treatment protocol, for 77.8% of all HPI alarms the appropriate intervention was performed. In light of the protocol, it is most likely that the intervention group was administered with less crystalloid fluid and more colloid fluid. It should be noted that the authors described that a lower HPI threshold of 80 was used to achieve early intervention (Schneck et al. 2020).

In addition, Wijnberge et al. performed a similar pilot RCT in which 68 patients were assigned to an HPI-guided treatment protocol or to standard care. The HPI-guided treatment group, which was consulted with HPI values >85, included treatment recommendations based on hemodynamic variables indicating problems in preload, afterload, or contractility. Through observation and comparison, it was found that time spent in hypotension (2.8% vs 10.3% of total procedure time, $P < 0.001$) was less, but no differences were observed in administered fluids or vasopressors. Fluid boluses were used more frequently in the intervention group than in the control group (16% vs 6%, $P < 0.001$). In contrast, phenylephrine (24% vs 19%, P ¼ 0.04) and ephedrine (14% vs 6%, $P < 0.001$) were used more frequently in the control group. These differences in treatment choice suggest a shift toward more frequent but fewer interventions and toward more frequent infusions in the intervention group, but no overall effect on total infusions and vasopressors (Wijnberge et al. 2020).

Apart from HPI, using arterial pressure waveform as the basis to predict hypotension with a machine learning algorithm is considered to be convincing. Hatib et al. proposed a model that relates a large set of features calculated from the arterial pressure waveform to the prediction of an impending hypotensive event (Hatib et al. 2018). This model employs machine learning to map the arterial pressure waveform features that serve to predict the hypotension. At the same time, it adopts logistic regression as the classification method for prediction. After training, the algorithm output can predict whether the patient has a tendency to develop hypotension. When the algorithm output is low, the likelihood of a hypotensive event is also low, and the time interval until the event occurs tends to be longer. Conversely, when the algorithm output is high, the likelihood of a hypotensive event is higher and the time interval until the event occurs tends to be shorter.

Using the vast electronic bandwidth, Lee and colleagues demonstrate an example of deep learning applied to perioperative practice (Lee et al. 2021). Their study showed that a deep learning model can predict hypotension in real time 5 min, 10 min, and 15 min before hypotensive events based on biosignals obtained using routine invasive and noninvasive patient monitoring. The model performed well across different patients and procedure types. Also, similar to other machine learning models, the model performs better when using a combined signal rather than a single signal. Deep learning algorithms are increasingly being used to analyze biosignal waveforms to predict various types of medical conditions. In the model of LEE et al., the prediction of medical conditions is based on detecting changes and signs of biosignals caused by diseases, physiological conditions, or compensatory mechanisms. Unsupervised learning can benefit from detecting clinically undetectable and subtle changes that cannot be recognized by human vision. The model features unsupervised feature extraction from multiple heterogeneous biosignals (Lee et al. 2021).

Over the same period, in 2020, Cherifa et al. used the Super Learner (SL) algorithm to predict acute hypotensive episodes 10 min before their occurrence (Cherifa et al. 2020). Acute hypotensive episodes (AHE) refer to a fall in mean arterial pressure (MAP) <65 mmHg lasting at least 5 min, which are one of the most serious events in the intensive care unit as they are associated with adverse outcomes in critically ill patients. Anticipating AHE allows for adjusting the treatment to prepare for or shorten the duration of AHE; thus, reducing the risk of surgery. The authors utilized the SL algorithm, an ensemble machine learning algorithm, and specifically trained it to achieve the goal of predicting AHE 10 min in advance. Potential predictors include age, gender, type of care unit, severity scores, and time-evolving features such as mechanical ventilation, vasopressors, or sedative drugs, as well as features extracted from physiological signals. The algorithm was trained on the MIMIC II dataset (Medical Information Mart for Intensive Care). An external validation was carried out using a dataset from the Lariboisière Hospital in Paris and its internal validation was based on the area under the receiver operating characteristic curve (AUROC) and the Brier score (BS). The study includes 1151 candidates, with 1 single random period per patient, the SL algorithm with Haar wavelets transform preprocessing was associated with an AUROC of 0.929 (95% confidence interval [CI], 0.899–0.958) and a BS of 0.08. SL with Haar wavelets transform preprocessing was associated with an AUROC of 0.89 (95% CI, 0.886–0.895) and a BS of 0.11 (Cherifa et al. 2020). The result shows that the SL algorithm shows good performance in predicting AHE 10 min in advance. It allows a valid, robust, and rapid assessment of the risk of hypotension, opening the way for routine use.

3 Artificial Intelligence in Prediction for Intraoperative Hypoxemia

Hypoxemia, also called low arterial oxygen tension, is an undesired physiological condition that can cause serious harm to patients when this condition occurs during general anesthesia and surgery (Dunham et al. 2014). Hypoxemia is associated with cardiac arrest, cardiac arrhythmias, postoperative infections and impaired wound healing, cognitive impairment and delirium, and cerebral ischemia through a number of metabolic pathways. Although oxygen saturation (SpO_2) is monitored continuously during general and regional anesthesia using pulse oximetry, hypoxemia can neither be reliably predicted nor prevented at a future time point. Real-time oxygen monitoring via pulse oximetry only allows the anesthesiologist to take reactive action to minimize the duration of hypoxemic episodes after they occur. According to the relevant guidelines, although decision support systems that process electronic medical record data can help improve the management of hypoxemia after it occurs, they do not reverse the essential problem of reactive management rather than predictive response. If hypoxemia can be predicted or anticipated before it occurs, then anesthesiologists can act to proactively prevent hypoxemia and minimize harm to patients.

Although anesthesiologists make every effort to avoid intraoperative hypoxemia, it is currently not possible to reliably predict future intraoperative hypoxemia. Scott et al. report the development and testing of a machine learning-based system that predicts the risk of hypoxemia and provides an explanation of risk factors in real time during general anesthesia. The system, trained on minute-by-minute data from electronic medical records of over 50,000 procedures, improved anesthesiologists' performance by providing interpretable hypoxemia risks and contributing factors. The interpretation of predictions is broadly consistent with the literature and the anesthesiologist's prior knowledge. The findings suggest that if anesthesiologists are currently able to predict 15% of hypoxemic events, with the help of the system their predictive ability could be improved to 30%, a large portion of which may benefit from early intervention as it relates to modifiable factors. The system can help understand the risk of hypoxemia during anesthesia care by providing general insight into the exact variability of risk due to certain characteristics of the patient or procedure (Lundberg et al. 2018).

According to different anesthesia contexts, there are studies exploring the combination of AI and medical treatment. Geng et al. assess the value of an artificial neural network (ANN) model in predicting hypoxemia during sedation for gastrointestinal endoscopy (Geng et al. 2019). Using propofol sedation during anesthesiologist-directed endoscopic procedures improves patient comfort and guarantees the smooth performance of endoscopic procedures. However, propofol may cause sedation-related complications because it exacerbates airway collapse and lowers the threshold for upper airway obstruction and hypoxemia. Therefore, early identification of patients at high risk for hypoxemia before endoscopy can help physicians take prompt and active interventions (e.g., chin lift, positive pressure ventilation, and tracheal intubation). In complex, multidimensional, and nonlinear relationships between predictors and prognosis, artificial neural networks can be used to predict clinical outcomes. Iterations and tours were set to 500 for the ANN in the study. A convergence criterion of 0.00001 was selected along with an overfit penalty of 0.001. The output of the ANN was converted to a range of 0–1; hypoxemia was predicted if the output was greater than or equal to 0.5. Receiver operating characteristic (ROC) curves were constructed and the area under the receiver operating characteristic curve (AUC) was used to assess the performance of the ANN model and other predictions. The criterion for excellent performance was an AUC above 0.8. This study concluded that the ANN model, built on three variables (BMI, habitual snoring, and neck circumference), is a useful tool for predicting hypoxemia during endoscopy (Geng et al. 2019).

References

Cherifa M, Blet A, Chambaz A, Gayat E, Resche-Rigon M, Pirracchio R. Prediction of an acute hypotensive episode during an ICU hospitalization with a super learner machine-learning algorithm. Anesth Analg. 2020;130(5):1157–66. https://doi.org/10.1213/ANE.0000000000004539.

Davies SJ, Vistisen ST, Jian Z, Hatib F, Scheeren TWL. Ability of an arterial waveform analysis-derived hypotension prediction index to predict future hypotensive events in surgical patients. Anesth Analg. 2020;130:352e359.

Dunham CM, Hileman BM, Hutchinson AE, Chance EA, Huang GS. Perioperative hypoxemia is common with horizontal positioning during general anesthesia and is associated with major adverse outcomes: a retrospective study of consecutive patients. BMC Anesthesiol. 2014;14:43.

Geng W, Tang H, Sharma A, Zhao Y, Yan Y, Hong W. An artificial neural network model for prediction of hypoxemia during sedation for gastrointestinal endoscopy. J Int Med Res. 2019;47(5):2097–103. https://doi.org/10.1177/0300060519834459. Epub 2019 Mar 26.

Hatib F, Jian Z, Buddi S, Lee C, Settels J, Sibert K, Rinehart J, Cannesson M. Machine-learning algorithm to predict hypotension based on high-fidelity arterial pressure waveform analysis. Anesthesiology. 2018;129(4):663–74. https://doi.org/10.1097/ALN.0000000000002300.

Kang AR, Lee J, Jung W, Lee M, Park SY, Woo J, et al. Development of a prediction model for hypotension after induction of anesthesia using machine learning. PLoS One. 2020;15(4):e0231172. https://doi.org/10.1371/journal.pone.0231172.

Lee S, Lee HC, Chu YS, Song SW, Ahn GJ, Lee H, Yang S, Koh SB. Deep learning models for the prediction of intraoperative hypotension. Br J Anaesth. 2021;126(4):808–17. https://doi.org/10.1016/j.bja.2020.12.035. Epub 2021 Feb 6.

Lundberg SM, Nair B, Vavilala MS, Horibe M, Eisses MJ, Adams T, Liston DE, Low DK, Newman SF, Kim J, Lee SI. Explainable machine-learning predictions for the prevention of hypoxaemia during surgery. Nat Biomed Eng. 2018;2(10):749–60. https://doi.org/10.1038/s41551-018-0304-0. Epub 2018 Oct 10.

Radhakrishnan S, Nair SG, Isaac J. Analysis of parameters affecting blood oxygen saturation and modeling of fuzzy logic system for inspired oxygen prediction. Comput Methods Prog Biomed. 2019;176:43–9. https://doi.org/10.1016/j.cmpb.2019.04.014. Epub 2019 Apr 30

Ranucci M, Barile L, Ambrogi F, Pistuddi V. Discrimination and calibration properties of the hypotension probability indicator during cardiac and vascular surgery. Minerva Anestesiol. 2019;85:724e730.

Schneck E, Schulte D, Habig L, et al. Hypotension prediction index based protocolized haemodynamic management reduces the incidence and duration of intraoperative hypotension in primary total hip arthroplasty: a single centre feasibility randomised blinded prospective interventional trial. J Clin Monit Comput. 2020;34:1149e1158.

Van der Ven WH, Veelo DP, Wijnberge M, van der Ster BJP, Vlaar APJ, Geerts BF. One of the first validations of an artificial intelligence algorithm for clinical use: the impact on intraoperative hypotension prediction and clinical decision-making. Surgery. 2021;169(6):1300–3. https://doi.org/10.1016/j.surg.2020.09.041. Epub 2020 Dec 11.

Wijnberge M, Geerts BF, Hol L, et al. Effect of a machine learning-derived early warning system for intraoperative hypotension vs standard care on depth and duration of intraoperative hypotension during elective noncardiac surgery: the HYPE randomized clinical trial. JAMA. 2020;323:1052e1060.

Application of Artificial Intelligence in ICU Management

Ningning Ji

Since 2011, with the rapid advancement of natural language processing and image analysis technologies, artificial intelligence (AI) technology, with deep learning as the main technology, has shown great potential in many fields such as disease diagnosis, image recognition and drug development, and has become an important tool to promote the change of medical industry. ICUs are data-intensive, technology-intensive, and knowledge-intensive, and are an important place for information technology applications, whose integration with AI is gradually entering the application stage as data availability increases and information sharing level improves. More and more scholars started to develop and introduce intelligent decision support systems, risk alert systems, and smart devices in ICUs to improve ICU healthcare practice and promote ICU healthcare service innovation.

1 AI in Decision-Making Support

ICU staffs need to make a comprehensive analysis of patient conditions in a short period of time, and this decision-making process requires solid theoretical knowledge and rich clinical experience. With the development of machine learning, especially deep learning and natural language processing, AI technologies can rapidly and comprehensively analyze patient data to derive individualized patient care plans and effectively assist healthcare professionals in decision-making. The algorithm developed by Laures et al. based on evidence can help healthcare professionals in intensive care units to select the most appropriate pain assessment method for their patients and improve pain assessment practices (Laures et al. 2021). AI technologies can assist and support healthcare professionals in decision-making, facilitate the clinical application of best evidence, and bring homogenization, standardization, and science to the healthcare delivery process.

1.1 Clinical Decision Support System

Researchers have developed a hardware system called clinical decision support system (CDSS) with the growing popularity of AIMS, which analyzes a comprehensive database using machine learning. The system provides anesthesiologists with timely decision aids and helps eliminate errors. Through data transformations, filtering, and filling in gaps, CDSS transforms and categorizes AIMS data into usable data. Based on the set decision rules, the decision processor

N. Ji (✉)
Department of Anesthesiology, Shanghai Ninth People's Hospital, Shanghai Jiao Tong University School of Medicine, Shanghai, China

M. Xia, H. Jiang (eds.), *Artificial Intelligence in Anesthesiology*,
https://doi.org/10.1007/978-981-99-5925-9_7

determines whether to notify or to alert AIMS, and on the basis of the alert prompts, anesthesiologists decide autonomously how the treatment plan should proceed.

Clinical culture, processes, workflows, and professional norms all play a role in the success of CDSS implementation. The implementation of CDSS is challenging from a number of perspectives, including system, organizational, and human factors. Due to the complexity of the healthcare process, it is difficult to ensure that improving one aspect of it does not lead to unintended consequences in another.

The scope of CDSS is also beyond that of an information technology tool, which can pose a challenge for adoption. Clinical practice is integrated with a paradigm of evidence-based practice. CDSS can often challenge deeply ingrained beliefs about professional autonomy and authority hierarchies in the clinical setting, leaving scientists skeptical of its use. A number of studies have examined the technical appropriateness and user experience of CDSS, but very few have explored how perceptions are influenced by the characteristics of end users.

Some scholars have developed corresponding CDSSs for glucose management (Lipton et al. 2011), temperature management (Fortier et al. 2006), and potassium regulation management (Hoekstra et al. 2010) of ICU patients, which improve the accuracy of data recording and provide nurses with immediate and appropriate decision-making solutions in the form of alerts, reminders, and recommendations. It is suggested that although CDSS can help healthcare providers to provide different decision-making options for different patients' conditions, it is important not to over-rely on the decision-making system and neglect the observation of patients' conditions, leading to poor decision-making.

In ICU, CDSS can also be applied to airway management. Lyerla found that evidence of bedhead elevation angle of mechanically ventilated patients was formed into a nursing decision support system, and a support system for protective ventilation strategies for mechanical ventilation in the ICU was designed, which could remind nurses to implement preventive measures to reduce the occurrence of ventilator-associated pneumonia (Frank 2008). Hu designed and implemented a CDSS for ventilator-associated pneumonia in ICU with rich decision dimensions, and fast decision speed and validated the decision accuracy of the system in actual clinical data, which provided a decision basis for the prevention, diagnosis, and treatment of ventilator-associated pneumonia in ICU and improved the decision efficiency of healthcare workers (Hu 2017).

2 AI in the Risk Alert

The ICU is equipped with a variety of advanced monitoring devices to help ICU staffs obtain data on multiple aspects of the patient's condition in order to detect early dynamic changes. In the early days, ICU nurses were required to monitor patients closely at the bedside in real time to determine possible changes in condition and care problems based on a large amount of raw data, which had limitations in terms of manpower and efficiency. Scholars have begun to try to use AI technology to transform the large amount of real-time monitoring data generated in the ICU into valuable medical information and to achieve intelligent risk alert. A Japanese hospital used machine learning based on the random forest algorithm to predict the pain level of patients based on parameters such as vital signs, age, and sedation level (Kobayashi et al. 2021). The results showed that the use of machine learning could objectively, continuously, and semi-automatically assess the pain experienced by ICU patients with an accuracy rate of 85.3%, which not only helped to optimize analgesic management but also had some value in promoting patient recovery. Sotoodeh et al. (2021) used unstructured data related to stress injury in electronic medical records, especially nursing records, to build predictive models using algorithms such as random forest and neural networks, which can predict the risk of a stress injury in advance and assist in intervention timing decisions. Shi et al. (2018) invented an intelligent sputum sound analysis system that automatically identifies sputum deposition in mechanically ventilated patients in the ICU and provides alerts when patients have excessive sputum accumulation. In addition, several AI-based predictive models have been developed in recent years, including sepsis prediction, risk of rebleeding in patients with gastrointestinal bleeding, ventilator extubation failure prediction, and human–machine confrontation prediction. By predicting the risk of various events and alerting ICU staffs to take precautionary measures, these models reduce the workload and stress of nurses while ensuring patient safety.

2.1 Monitoring Vital Signs

Continuous vital sign monitoring techniques are commonly used in patients with deteriorating conditions or those considered to be at high risk of deterioration. Early identification of signs of deterioration and clinical intervention can reduce the occurrence of adverse patient events. False alarms are a significant problem during continuous monitoring, and technical issues such as electromagnetic interference and wire dislodgement explain the false alarms. Wearable vital sign monitoring devices are a new type of device that is portable and performs continuous vital sign monitoring without the patient being connected to the device by wires, which reduces the number of false alarms caused by technical aspects to a certain extent. Another important reason for generating false alarms is the lack of personalized settings for patients, and the application of machine learning makes personalized medicine a possibility. Ostojic et al. intelligently analyzed physiological monitoring and reduced false alarm rates by combining brain oximetry data with machine learning algorithms (Ostojic et al. 2020). Mousavi et al. further used convolutional neural networks to automatically extract data, and this method in the task of reducing virtual alarms achieved better results with a sensitivity of 93.88% and a specificity of 92.05% for alarm classification (Mousavi et al. 2020). Ansari et al. used machine learning methods to effectively reduce the incidence of false arrhythmia alarms, which also provides more evidence for the application of machine learning to vital sign monitoring techniques (Ansari et al. 2016).

2.2 Monitoring Subtle Activity

ICU patients may experience subtle and sudden responses after a period of unconsciousness, such as finger and toe movements or blinking, which are unpredictable and difficult to identify (Magi and Prasad 2020). Traditional human observation methods are inefficient and may miss the patient's minute movements. A non-invasive mobility sensor (NIMS) designed by Reiter et al. can locate, track, and identify the person and determine the highest level of movement by predicting the patient's posture. Magi et al. developed a novel hand monitoring system that uses image processing and deep learning to monitor ICU patients in real time, categorizing patients' hands as "normal" or "abnormal" (Magi and Prasad 2020). The latter indicates that the patient has hand activity, at which point the system alerts the doctor or nurse with an alarm so that the patient can be treated as soon as possible. However, this system is currently only applicable to hand observation and has not been extended to whole-body monitoring.

2.3 Early Recognition of Delirium

Delirium is an acute disorder of consciousness and cognitive function, and studies have shown that 23.06–30.80% of patients in the ICU develop delirium. With pervasive sensing technology and AI, Davoudi et al. used sensors and cameras to capture data and found significant differences in facial expressions, limb movements, and postural functional status between delirious and non-delirious patients after analysis (Davoudi et al. 2019). Delirium in patients may be related to autonomic instability, which can be assessed by heart rate variability. Based on the above hypothesis, Oh et al. developed a delirium prediction model using heart rate variability and machine learning methods, which has a certain degree of confidence and validity (Oh et al. 2018). Mikalsen et al. developed an anchor word-based delirium recognition model using a consistent clustering algorithm and a t-distributed stochastic neighbor embedding algorithm by automatically reading medical records by computer (Mikalsen et al. 2017). The area under the accuracy rate curve was 0.96, but the correct rate of this model for diagnosing delirium was related to the quality of the electronic medical record text, and further verification of the related sensitivity and specificity is needed.

2.4 Prediction of Mortality Risk

Studies have reported high in-hospital mortality rates for patients in the ICU, ranging from 6.7% to 44.0% worldwide (Weigl et al. 2017, 2018). In clinical practice, physicians need to take into account the medical history, physical examination, and trends in vital signs when assessing patients' conditions and making clinical decisions, which is a huge workload. Especially for ICU patients, an accurate, reliable, and convenient assessment can help physicians to make decisions and take timely treatment measures. At present, ICU mostly uses the scoring system for mortality assessment. It is significant to further protect the life safety of ICU patients if a prediction model can be established using objective indicators to simplify and automate the assessment method and obtain more accurate and reliable assessment results.

In recent years, machine learning, as an important branch of AI, has been widely used in the field of healthcare, and has great potential in mining and processing medical data to make up for the shortcomings of linear models. Lin (2018) constructed a prediction model for the risk of in-hospital death in patients with acute renal impairment in ICU based on the support vector machine approach and compared its prediction performance with that of a simplified acute physiological score, after that, concluded that the SVM model presented better prediction performance. The study mentioned above was conducted only for patients with acute renal impairment in the ICU and was not applicable to all ICU inpatients. The metric variables used were the same as the simplified acute physiology score, and fewer metrics were included in the study. For the deep learning model long short-term memory (LSTM) artificial neural network and its derivative gated recurrent unit (GRU), better AUCROC and AUC-PR were achieved in predicting mortality in ICU patients. However, LSTM and GRU have disadvantages such as computationally large, time consuming, high hardware requirements, and gradient disappearance, making it difficult to process and apply large data for clinical dissemination. Note that the mechanism mimics the data processing mode of the human brain and is currently combined with LSTM or other deep learning methods to improve computational efficiency or interpretability (Yu et al. 2020). However, inefficiency, a limitation of the method itself, is still unavoidable.

Deng et al. (2022) introduced a classification algorithm, support vector machine (SVM) method, which shows unique advantages in solving finite samples, nonlinear and high-dimensional problems. It has a perfect mathematical form with intuitive geometric interpretation, and unlike the structural design of neural networks, it does not depend on the designer's empirical and a priori knowledge, has few artificially set parameters, is easy to use, and therefore has a better generalization capability. The core idea of using kernel functions to map complex classification problems into linearly differentiable problems cleverly solves the problem of "curse of dimensionality."

3 AI in Assistance of Nurses' Work

Due to the special nature of ICU patients and the closed environment, ICU nurses are the main focus of all activities. Studies have shown that the workload of ICU nurses is significantly higher than that of nurses in general wards, and devices developed based on AI technology can assist or replace nurses to complete some low-tech repetitive tasks so that nurses can devote more time and energy to patient care. Yuan et al. developed an intelligent suction robot with a roller drive, which was tested to have a success rate of ≥95% in delivering and withdrawing suction tubes, and is expected to replace traditional suction operations in the future (Yuan et al. 2020). Peine et al. developed and evaluated a new non-contact visual recognition system to identify and track the use of medical consumables in the ICU through deep learning methods, at the same time, to automatically register them in hospital electronic records (Peine et al. 2019). The system automatically registers the hospital's electronic records and predicts the number of consumables used, enabling intelligent management of consumables. The application of intelligent devices can assist or replace nurses in completing some repetitive curing and simple operations, alleviate the current severe situation of global nursing human resources shortage, and promote the intelligent development of the nursing model.

3.1 Controlling the Risk of Infection

Hospital-acquired infections affect patient morbidity, mortality and quality of life, and are an important public health issue. Proper and effective hand hygiene can reduce the occurrence of hospital-acquired infections, but related studies have shown that ICU nurses have low awareness of hand hygiene. Myo is an electronic wearable device designed for gesture control, which builds an effective gesture recognition algorithm through electromyography, acceleration, and rotation data (Kutafina et al. 2015). Pan et al. combined IoT technology, positioning technology, and behavior recognition technology to design a monitoring system that records nurses' actions through a badge and uses indicator lights and warning tones to remind nurses of hand hygiene before and after they enter and exit dangerously infected areas, and the results showed that the effective hand washing rate of nurses increased by 43.3% after applying the new system compared with that before implementation (Pan et al. 2020). This finding is supported by the studies of Wang et al. (2021) and Zhong et al. (2021), which suggest that the real-time monitoring and reminder function has some merit in improving hand hygiene among healthcare workers. Effective and continuous environmental cleaning and disinfection are also key to reducing hospital-acquired infections, and disinfection service robots can be used to sterilize microorganisms by producing dry mist that is invisible to the naked eye and adheres to the surface. The 3D sensor smart toothbrush collects and analyzes data on brushing accuracy, duration, and frequency to provide customized recommendations, displaying areas missed by brushing on a tooth distribution diagram.

3.2 Simplifying the Nursing Process

Patient handling is a common operation in clinical nursing, which not only consumes nurses' physical strength but also easily causes skeletal muscle injury in the long run. Wang et al. invented a modular symmetrical transfer nursing robot, which can realize the transfer of patients between hospital beds and stretcher carts. He et al. designed a combined nursing bed (He 2016), which can automatically convert hospital beds into wheelchairs during operation. An item transfer robot is another technological innovation that streamlines the nursing process. With sensors, a wireless network, and a central hospital system, the robot can execute commands as required. The new coronavirus pneumonia epidemic is driving the rapid development of the robotics industry. During the COVID-19 outbreak, intelligent robots perform activities such as delivering meals and medications according to a preset route, effectively avoiding direct human contact and cutting off the spread of the virus at the source. The robots can also help nurses obtain supplies and deliver them to preset locations.

4 AI in Remote Intensive Care

Remote intensive care is a new medical model that provides remote healthcare for patients in off-site locations with the help of advanced information technology and equipment to achieve the sharing of quality medical resources. Studies have shown that remote intensive care has positive effects in the prevention and management of venous thromboembolism, catheter-associated bloodstream infections, and ventilator-associated pneumonia, but it is not yet commonly practiced. Some foreign hospitals use an intelligent color coding system to classify the risk of patients in the remote monitoring ward, therefore, remotely alert ICU nurses to changes in patients' conditions through alarms and prioritize their work, effectively reducing the incidence of adverse events. The development of remote intensive care in China is still in its infancy, and most hospitals are committed to applying network systems for remote consultation. The remote medicine platform of Karamay Central Hospital of Xinjiang was put into use in 2017 (Lai et al. 2018), which has improved medical technology diagnosis and treatment while saving transfer costs and reducing the financial burden for patients' families. After the outbreak of COVID-19, the advantages of remote critical care have become increasingly evident. Through the application of medical-assisted robots, big data analysis, cloud platforms, remote medicine, and intelligent monitoring, the risk of cross-regional transmission of personnel is reduced while completing medical services, allowing limited medical resources to maximize their value.

5 Summary

ICU is an area where management of quality, efficiency, and accuracy is required. It surely poses a strict demand on ICU staff's work, at the same time, it suggests the possibility of implementing AI into ICU management. From the discussion in this chapter, it can be found that AI can support ICU management in decision-making, risk alert, the assistance of nurses' work, and remote intensive care. AI has already taken an important role in ICU management, and there are further ways of application that remain to be discovered, which brings numerous topics for future studies in this field.

References

Ansari S, Belle A, Ghanbari H, Salamango M, Najarian K. Suppression of false arrhythmia alarms in the ICU: a machine learning approach. Physiol Meas. 2016;37(8):1186–203.

Davoudi A, Malhotra KR, Shickel B, Siegel S, Williams S, Ruppert M, et al. Intelligent ICU for autonomous patient monitoring using pervasive sensing and deep learning. Sci Rep. 2019;9(1):8020.

Deng P, Chen Y-W, Li Y-J, Yang Z-Y, Zhong K-H, Zhang J, Lu K-Z, Yi B. Prediction of in-hospital mortality risk in intensive care unit with support vector machine. J Army Med Univ. 2022;44(17):1764–9.

Fortier P, Michel H, Sarangarajan B, Dluhy N, Oneill E. A computerized decision support aid for critical care novice nursing. In: Proceedings of the 38th annual Hawaii international conference on system sciences, vol. 2006; 2006. p. 444–8.

He H-Z. Combined nursing bed: USA; 2016. p. 9295596.2016-03-29.

Hoekstra M, Vogelzang M, Drost JT, Janse M, Loef BG, van der Horst ICC, et al. Implementation and evaluation of a nurse-centered computerized potassium regulation protocol in the intensive care unit – a before and after analysis. BMC Med Inform Decis Mak. 2010;10(1):5.

Hu Y. Design and implementation of a clinical decision support system for ventilator-associated pneumonia in the ICU [D]. Shanghai: Shanghai Jiaotong University; 2017.

Kobayashi N, Shiga T, Ikumi S, Watanabe K, Murakami H, Yamauchi M. Semi-automated tracking of pain in critical care patients using artificial intelligence: a retrospective observational study. Sci Rep. 2021;11(1):5229.

Kutafina E, Laukamp D, Jonas SM. Wearable sensors in medical education: supporting hand hygiene training with a forearm EMG. Stud Health Technol Inform. 2015;211:286–91.

Lai Y-C, Ye Z, Xia T. The innovative design and application of e-ICU system based on Internet + remote intensive care. China Digit Med. 2018; 13(7): 43–45.

Laures EL, Bruene D, Fayram LR, Houston A, Kephart K, Merrifield E, et al. Pediatric pain assessment in the intensive care unit: an evidence-based algorithm. Pain Manag Nurs. 2021;22(3):260–7.

Lin K. Application of support vector machine in predicting in-hospital mortality risk of patients with acute kidney injury in ICU. J Peking Univ. 2018;50(2):239–44.

Lipton JA, Barendse RJ, Schinkel AFL, Akkerhuis KM, Simoons ML, Sijbrands EJG. Impact of an alerting clinical decision support system for glucose control on protocol compliance and glycemic control in the intensive cardiac care unit. Diabetes Technol Ther. 2011;13(3):343–9.

Frank L. Design and implementation of a nursing clinical decision support system to promote guideline adherence. Comput Inform Nurs. 2008;26(4):227–33.

Magi N, Prasad BG. Activity monitoring for ICU patients using deep learning and image processing. SN Comput Sci. 2020; 1(3): 123.

Mikalsen KØ, Soguero-Ruiz C, Jensen K, Hindberg K, Gran M, Revhaug A, et al. Using anchors from free text in electronic health records to diagnose postoperative delirium. Comput Methods Prog Biomed. 2017;152:105–14.

Mousavi S, Fotoohinasab A, Afghah F. Single-modal and multi-modal false arrhythmia alarm reduction using attention-based convolutional and recurrent neural networks. PLoS One. 2020;15(1):e0226990.

Oh J, Cho D, Park J, Na SH, Kim J, Heo J, et al. Prediction and early detection of delirium in the intensive care unit by using heart rate variability and machine learning. Physiol Meas. 2018;39(3):035004.

Ostojic D, Guglielmini S, Moser V, Fauchère JC, Bucher HU, Bassler D, et al. Reducing false alarm rates in neonatal intensive care: a new machine learning approach. Adv Exp Med Biol. 2020;1232:285–90.

Pan X-D, Xie W-W, Chen M-J, Yu F-F. Application of smart control hand hygiene IoT system in ICU nurses' hand hygiene management. J Tradit Chin Med Manag. 2020;28(17):55–6.

Peine A, Hallawa A, Schöffski O, Dartmann G, Fazlic LB, Schmeink A, et al. A deep learning approach for managing medical consumable materials in intensive care units via convolutional neural networks: technical proof-of-concept study. JMIR Med Inform. 2019;7(4):e14806.

Shi Y, Wang G, Niu J, Zhang Q, Cai M, Sun B, et al. Classification of sputum sounds using artificial neural network and wavelet transform. Int J Biol Sci. 2018;14(8):938–45.

Sotoodeh M, Gero ZH, Zhang W, Hertzberg VS, Ho JC. Pressure ulcer injury in unstructured clinical notes: detection and interpretation [Internet]. AMIA Annu Symp Proc. 2021;2020:1160–9. [cited 2023Feb9]. https://www.ncbi.nlm.nih.gov/pmc/articles/PMC8075497/.

Wang L-Q, Yu L, Li X-Y, Li M, He X-M. Evaluation of hand hygiene effectiveness of real-time monitoring intervention for medical staff in critical care medicine. Chin J of Nosocomiol. 2021;31(5):796–800.

Weigl W, Adamski J, Goryński P, Kański A, Hultström M. Mortality rate is higher in polish intensive care units than in other European countries. Intensive Care Med. 2017;43(9):1430–2.

Weigl W, Adamski J, Goryński P, Kański A, Hultström M. ICU mortality and variables associated with ICU survival in Poland. Eur J Anaesthesiol. 2018;35(12):949–54.

Yu R, Zheng Y, Zhang R, Jiang Y, Poon CC. Using a multi-task recurrent neural network with attention mechanisms to predict hospital mortality of patients. IEEE J Biomed Health Inform. 2020;24(2):486–92.

Yuan L-R, Tan W-J, Zhu H-Y, et al. Experimental study on safety and effectiveness of intelligent sputum-sucking robot. Clin Res Pract. 2020;5(17):5–8.

Zhong X, Wang D-L, Xiao L-H, Mo L-F, Wu Q-F, Chen Y-W, et al. Comparison of two electronic hand hygiene monitoring systems in promoting hand hygiene of healthcare workers in the intensive care unit. BMC Infect Dis. 2021;21(1):50.

Artificial Intelligence in Prediction and Management of PONV

Ming Xia

Even with the development of new anesthetic agents and techniques, the incidence of postoperative nausea and vomiting (PONV) still remains at about 30%. PONV may cause suture rupture, wound dehiscence, pulmonary aspiration, bleeding, dehydration, and electrolyte disturbance. Although anti-emetic prophylaxis can be helpful, routine efforts are generally contraindicated by cost and side effects of anti-emetics. In order to identify patients who would benefit from prophylactic anti-emetics, by now, researchers have been developing or verifying the predictive models for PONV. This chapter will review and analyze these models and provide useful suggestions for practice and future researches.

1 Guidelines for the Prediction and Management of PONV

1.1 Incidence of Postoperative Nausea and Vomiting and Its Adverse Effects

The incidence of postoperative nausea and vomiting (PONV) is 30% in general surgical patients and up to 80% in high-risk patients. PONV occurs mostly 24–48 h after surgery, and a few can last until 3–5 days after surgery (Echeverria-Villalobos et al. 2022).

PONV may cause patients to experience different degrees of pain, including water and electrolyte balance disorders, wound dehiscence, incisional hernia formation, misinhalation, and aspiration pneumonia, thereby reducing patient satisfaction, prolonging hospitalization time, and increasing medical costs.

1.2 Risk Factors of PONV

1.2.1 Patient Factors

Female, PONV and/or motion sickness history, non-smoking, age less than 50 years. Risk factors for the occurrence of PONV in children include age 3 years and older, history of POV/PONV/sickness, family history of POV/PONV, post-pubertal females; strabismus surgery, adenotonsillectomy or otoplasty, surgery time 30 min and more, intraoperative use of inhalational anesthetics, anticholinergics; postoperative use of long-acting opioids (Veiga-Gil et al. 2017; Apfel et al. 2012; Kovac 2021).

1.2.2 Anesthetic Factors

The risk of PONV caused by inhaled anesthetics such as nitrous oxide depends on the duration of

M. Xia (✉)
Department of Anesthesiology, Shanghai Ninth People's Hospital, Shanghai Jiao Tong University School of Medicine, Shanghai, China
e-mail: xiaming1980@xzhmu.edu.cn

M. Xia, H. Jiang (eds.), *Artificial Intelligence in Anesthesiology*,
https://doi.org/10.1007/978-981-99-5925-9_8

surgery. Postoperative opioids, thiopental sodium, etomidate, ketamine, tramadol, etc., also increase the incidence of PONV. Insufficient volume increases the incidence of PONV. Propofol TIVA, multimodal analgesia, regional block anesthesia, and opioid dosage reduction reduce the incidence of PONV. Accelerated recovery strategy proposed that fasting after midnight may increase the risk of PONV.

1.2.3 Surgical Factors

The long duration of surgery (>3 h) is associated with an increased risk of PONV. The incidence of PONV is higher in laparoscopic surgery, bariatric surgery, gynecological surgery, cholecystectomy, and other types of surgery.

Apfel designed a simple adult PONV risk score based on four major risk factors for PONV in adults: female, non-smoking, history of PONV and/or motion sickness, and postoperative opioid use: each factor is scored as 1, and those with scores of 0, 1, 2, 3, and 4 have a 10%, 20%, 40%, 60%, and 80% risk of PONV, respectively. The five main risk factors for postoperative discharge nausea and vomiting (PDNV) in adults were female, history of PONV, age under 50 years, use of opioids in PACU and history of nausea in PACU, with scores of 0, 1, 2, 3, 4, and 5, respectively, the risk of PDNV was 10%, 20%, 30%, 50%, 60% and 80%. The four main high-risk factors for PONV in children are surgery time ≥ 30 min, age 3 years and above, strabismus surgery, history of PONV or history of PONV in the immediate family with scores of 0, 1, 2, 3, and 4, the risk of PONV was 10%, 10%, 30%, 50%, and 70%, respectively (Gan et al. 2014; Horn et al. 2014).

1.3 PONV Scoring

Visual analog scoring method (VAS): 10 cm straightedge as a scale, one end is 0, indicating no nausea and vomiting, the other end is 10, indicating the most severe nausea and vomiting that is unbearable (1–4 for mild, 5–6 for moderate, 7–10 for severe).

1.4 The Occurrence Mechanism of PONV

The vomiting center is located in the ventral posterior pole area of the fourth ventricle (Area postrema) chemical trigger zone and above the nucleus of the solitary bundle, divided into the neuroreflex center and chemoreceptor trigger zone.

The neuroreflex center receives afferent stimuli from the cortex (visual, olfactory, gustatory), pharynx, gastrointestinal and inner ear vestibular tract, coronary artery, and chemoreceptor trigger zone. The chemical trigger band includes 5-HT3 receptors, 5-HT4 receptors, opioid receptors, cholinergic receptors, cannabinoid receptors, dopamine receptors, and a variety of other sites associated with nausea and vomiting.

The efferent nerves for nausea and vomiting include the vagus, sympathetic, and phrenic nerves.

1.5 Classification of Anti-emetic Drugs

Anti-emetic drugs can be classified according to their action sites: (1) acting in the cortex: benzodiazepines; (2) acting in the chemical trigger zone: phenothiazines (chlorpromazine, promethazine, and prochlorazide), butylphenols (haloperidol and haloperidol), 5-HT3 receptor antagonists (ondansetron, granisetron, toltesetron, azathioprine, dolasetron, and palonosetron), NK-1 receptor antagonists (aprepitant), benzamides, cannabinoids; (3) acting in the vomiting center: anti-dopaminergic drugs (amisulpride), antihistamines (benzosin and hydroxyzine), anticholinergics (scopolamine); (4) acting in the visceral afferent nerves: 5-HT_3 receptor antagonists, benzamides (metoclopramide); and (5) other: corticosteroids (dexamethasone, methylprednisolone).

1.5.1 Anti-dopaminergic Drugs

Amisulpride is an oral antipsychotic agent as a dopamine D_2 and D_3 receptor antagonist.

In patients who have been given non-antidopaminergic drugs to prevent PONV, amisulpride 10 mg is more effective compared to placebo for PONV. Amisulpride 5 mg was given before induction to prevent postoperative nausea and vomiting (Haber et al. 2021).

1.5.2 Anticholinergic Drugs

The mechanism of action of these drugs is to inhibit muscarinic-like cholinergic receptors and inhibit acetylcholine release. This class of drugs can block the impulse afferent to the vestibule, mainly used for the treatment of motion sickness, vertigo, viral otitis media, Meniere's disease, and tumor-induced nausea and vomiting. The main use of scopolamine patch to prevent and control PONV, side effects are dry mouth and blurred vision.

1.5.3 Antihistamines

Histamine receptors can be divided into H_1, H_2, and H_3 three types. H_1 receptors and allergic, inflammatory reactions related to H_2 receptors and gastric acid secretion, H_3 receptors and histamine release related. The recommended dose of diphenhydramine is 1 mg/kg for sedation. Promethazine can be effective in the treatment of PONV, 6.25 mg dose is effective, and the sedative effect is small (Athavale et al. 2020).

1.5.4 Butylphenols

Small doses of haloperidol (0.625–1.25 mg) can effectively prevent PONV, and ondansetron 4 mg effect is similar. Flupirtide may lead to QT interval prolongation and tip-twisting ventricular tachycardia by the US FDA black box warning, but many scholars and literature that such complications are time- and dose-dependent, mainly seen in antipsychotic weeks or months of continuous use, and small doses applied to PONV is safe, in adults using low doses of this product on the QT interval effect with Ondansetron and placebo no difference, but also suggests that in the prevention and treatment of PONV should avoid the use of high doses of this product or with other drugs that can prolong the QT interval, has proved that even in very small doses (10–15 μg/kg), also have anti-emetic effect (Elvir-Lazo et al. 2020). While increasing the dose enhances the anti-emetic effect, it also poses the risk of increased side effects such as sedation and extrapyramidal symptoms. Haloperidol is recommended as an alternative to haloperidol, 0.5–2 mg sedation or intramuscular injection has a good preventive effect on PONV and can be administered after induction or before the end of surgery, side effects include QT prolongation, similar to 5-HT_3 receptor antagonists.

1.5.5 Glucocorticoids

Dexamethasone and methylprednisolone anti-vomiting mechanism is still unclear. Since dexamethasone takes time to work, it should be administered at the beginning of the procedure, with the main concern being the possible increase of blood glucose in diabetic patients. Methylprednisolone 40 mg IV before induction may prevent postoperative nausea and vomiting (Shaikh et al. 2016).

1.5.6 Benzamide

Metoclopramide has central and peripheral dopamine receptor antagonism, also has an anti-serotonin effect, accelerates gastric emptying, inhibits gastric relaxation, and inhibits vomiting central chemoreceptor trigger band, most commonly used in gastric motility drugs and as adjuvant therapy for vomiting associated with antitumor chemotherapy, conventional dose of 10 mg has not been shown to have a preventive effect on PONV. A large sample of studies has shown that metoclopramide 25 mg or 50 mg in combination with dexamethasone 8 mg is better than dexamethasone 8 mg alone for the prevention of PONV, and such a high dose of metoclopramide significantly increases the complications of the extrapyramidal system.

1.5.7 5-HT_3 Receptor Antagonists

While 90% of 5-HT receptors are present in the gastrointestinal tract (gastrointestinal submucosa and intestinal chromophores), 1–2% of them are present in the central chemoreceptor trigger band (Mawe and Hoffman 2013).

Chemotherapy and postoperative emesis are associated with the activation of 5-HT_3 receptors in the submucosa of the gastrointestinal tract. It is recommended for the prophylaxis of PONV, especially in high-risk patients, and multiple therapeutic doses are not recommended if no effect is tried with another class of drugs. Studies have shown that the therapeutic effect and safety of all such drugs in the prevention of PONV do not differ. It has also been shown that low-dose granisetron (0.1 mg) compounded with 8 mg dexamethasone and ondansetron 4 mg compounded with dexamethasone 8 mg for the prevention of nausea and vomiting after hernia surgery can achieve excellent results of 94–97% within 2 h and 83–87% within 24 h after tracheal tube extraction (Ngo et al. 2019). The efficacy of ondansetron was similar to that of 4–8 mg dexamethasone and haloperidol. The efficacy of 0.3 mg IV ramosetron or 150 mg IV fosaprepitant were both superior to ondansetron.

The recommended dose of ondansetron for PONV is 4 mg, with the following side effects: headache (5–27%), diarrhea (<1–16%), constipation (<1–9%), fever (<1–8%), malaise or fatigue (0–13%), and increased liver enzymes (1–5%).

Toltestrone blocks 5-HT_3 receptors, and the main ring of the drug's structure is closest to 5-HT, making it more specific. This drug has a long half-life (8–12 h, ondansetron 3 h, granisetron 3.1–5.9 h) and is available in oral formulations.

Palonosetron is a second-generation, highly selective, high-affinity 5-HT_3 receptor antagonist with a half-life of 40 h. Compared to first-generation 5-HT_3 receptor antagonists, palonosetron has a similar structure to 5-HT and binds more readily to 5-HT_3 receptors. Studies have shown that 0.075 mg of palonosetron can effectively prevent the occurrence of PONV within 24 h after surgery, and its effect is similar to that of 4 mg of ondansetron (Yoo et al. 2018). Mainly metabolized by CYP2D6 enzyme, the clinical dose is not affected by age, liver and kidney functions, and has no significant effect on QT interval.

1.5.8 NK-1 Receptor Antagonist

Aprepitant has selectivity and high affinity for NK-1 receptors, low affinity for NK-2 and NK-3 receptors, and low affinity for dopamine receptors and 5-HT receptors. It exerts anti-emetic effects by binding to NK-1 receptors to block the action of substance P. Oral administration of 40 mg aprepitant 1–3 h before surgery can effectively prevent the occurrence of PONV within 48 h after surgery. The oral administration of 150 mg of casopitant before induction can also prevent postoperative nausea and vomiting.

1.5.9 Anesthetics

Small doses of propofol (20 mg) have anti-emetic effect, but the effect time is short. Studies have shown that midazolam 2 mg given 30 min before the end of surgery can effectively prevent PONV, and ondansetron 4 mg equivalent.

1.5.10 The Combination of Different Types of Anti-PONV Drugs

It can be used in combination to block a variety of central nervous system receptors; the efficacy is better than a single drug. In addition, due to the use of the lowest effective dose, the incidence of side effects of each drug is also reduced. Combinations of drugs are recommended for the prevention of PONV, such as 5-HT_3 receptor antagonists (ondansetron, palonosetron) + dexamethasone, 5-HT_3 receptor antagonists (ondansetron, palonosetron) + aprepitant, aprepitant + dexamethasone, 5-HT_3 receptor antagonists (ondansetron, palonosetron) + haloperidol, ondansetron + haloperidol, ondansetron + betahistine Ramosetron + gabapentin, dexamethasone + haloperidol, amisulpride + 1 non-dopaminergic anti-emetic, and dexamethasone + teicoplanin. 5-HT_3 receptor inhibitors work best when combined with haloperidol and dexamethasone (Law et al. 2003).

1.5.11 Acupoint Stimulation

Acupoint stimulation therapy may increase the release of beta-endorphin in vivo, activate adrenergic and noradrenergic nerve fibers to alter 5-HT3 transmission, and inhibit vagal nerve and gastric acid secretion to prevent and treat PONV. acupoint stimulation can be divided into invasive stimulation and noninvasive stimulation, invasive stimulation including acupuncture, electroacupuncture, acupoint injection, scar moxibustion, and buried thread, noninvasive stimulation including acupressure, transcutaneous electrical stimulation, indirect moxibustion, and ultralaser irradiation. Acupuncture points can be selected from the Nei Guan point (P6 point), the combination of the Nei Guan point with bilateral Hegu, Foot San Li, and San Yin Jiao points, and the auricular acupressure stimulation method (Acar 2016). Acupoint drug injections can be used for patients who are difficult or unsuitable for indwelling acupuncture, such as pediatric patients. For example, injection of 50% glucose 0.2 mL at the Neiguan acupoint in pediatric patients is comparable to haloperidol 10 μg/kg for the prevention and treatment of PONV (Elvir-Lazo et al. 2020).

1.5.12 Other Drugs

Preoperative gabapentin can reduce abdominal surgery patients with PONV. Hypnosis, ginger, small doses of naloxone, and other therapeutic measures have a certain anti-emetic effect.

1.6 Prevention and Control of PONV Principles

1.6.1 General Principles

Clinicians should determine the risk of patients to occur PONV, and patients at risk or above should be given effective drug prevention.

Removal of underlying causes, including appropriate preoperative fasting (not less than 6 h); preoperative insertion of coarse-caliber gastric tube single suction or continuous drainage for patients with gastrointestinal obstruction, intraoperative gastric distension patients should be placed in a large-caliber gastric tube before the end of surgery for a one-time suction, suction after removal of the gastric tube to reduce gastric tube irritation and reflux.

Epidural anesthesia, infiltration anesthesia, propofol intravenous anesthesia are conducive to reducing PONV. Dexmedetomidine given before skin incision can reduce the incidence of PONV. Short-acting opioids such as remifentanil, intraoperative rehydration in adequate amounts to avoid cerebral hypoxia ischemia, and using sugars instead of neostigmine to antagonize neuromuscular NSAIDs can significantly reduce the risk of PONV, but non-selective NSAIDs may be associated with gastrointestinal surgical anastomotic fistula and should be used with caution.

1.6.2 The Choice of Anti-vomiting Drugs and Administration Time

PONV clinical prevention and treatment effect is determined by the gold standard which is to achieve 24 h effective and completely without nausea and vomiting.

Different mechanisms of action of PONV drugs in combination with the prevention and treatment effect are better than a single drug, the effect of additive but not additive side effects. 5-HT_3 receptor inhibitors, dexamethasone and haloperidol or haloperidol are the most effective prevention of PONV and side effects of small drugs. Patients without PONV risk factors do not need prophylactic medication. For low- and intermediate-risk patients, one or two of these drugs can be used for prophylaxis. For high-risk patients, two to three drug combinations can be used for prevention.

The onset and duration of action of drugs should be considered for prophylaxis. Oral medications such as ondansetron, dolasetron, prochlorperazine, and aprepitant should be given 1–3 h before induction of anesthesia; intravenous anti-emetics should be administered before the end of surgery, but intravenous dexamethasone should be given after induction of anesthesia; and scopolamine patches should be given in the evening before surgery or 2–4 h before the start of surgery.

1.6.3 Anti-emetic Treatment for PONV

When persistent nausea and vomiting occur after the patient leaves the anesthesia recovery room, bedside investigations should first be performed to exclude drug stimulation or mechanical factors, including patient-controlled analgesia with morphine, blood drainage along the throat, or abdominal obstruction. After drug and mechanical factors are ruled out, anti-emetic therapy can be initiated.

If the patient has no prophylactic medication, treatment with a small dose of 5-HT_3 receptor antagonists should be started at the first presentation of PONV. The therapeutic dose of 5-HT_3 receptor antagonists is usually about 1/4 of the prophylactic dose, ondansetron 1 mg, dolasetron 12.5 mg, granisetron 0.1 mg, and toltesetron 0.5 mg, dexamethasone 2–4 mg, haloperidol 0.625 mg, or promethazine 6.25–12.5 mg (Theriot et al. 2022). Patients may be considered for treatment with propofol 20 mg by sedation when PONV occurs in the PACU.

If prophylactic medication has been administered, treatment should be switched to another type of drug. If PONV still occurs in patients after triple therapy (such as 5-HT3 receptor inhibitors, dexamethasone, and haloperidol or haloperidol) prophylaxis, these three drugs should not be repeated within 6 h of administration and should be replaced with other anti-emetics. If PONV occurs 6 h postoperatively, repeat administration of 5-HT_3 receptor antagonists and haloperidol or haloperidol may be considered at the same dose as before. Repeated application of dexamethasone is not recommended.

1.6.4 The Combination of Chinese and Western Medicines

Combination of anti-emetic drugs and transcutaneous electrical stimulation of acupuncture points or acupuncture, compared with a single method, can further reduce the incidence of nausea and vomiting, and reduce the incidence of anti-emetic side effects.

2 PONV Prediction Models

The purpose of constructing PONV prediction model is to screen PONV high-risk population so as to customize effective preventive measures. Some foreign studies have already designed their own PONV prediction models, such as Finland's Koivuranta et al. (1997) and Germany's Apfel et al. (1999) established prediction models as Risk = 1 ÷ [1 + exp. (−2.21 + 0.93 × female + 0. 82 × PONV history + 0.59 × history of motion sickness + 0.61 × non-smoking status + 0.75 × operation time over 60 min)] and Risk = 1 ÷ [1 + exp. (−2.28 + 1.27 × female + 0. 65 × PONV history + 0.72 × non-smoking status + 0.78 × postoperative opioid application)], the AUCs of the ROC curves were 0.72 and 0.75, respectively. But Van Den Bosch et al. in the Netherlands validated the predictive efficacy of these two prediction models. Apfel et al. (van den Bosch et al. 2005) also validated several different PONV prediction models in their own population and found that the AUC was only 0.61–0.71 (Apfel et al. 1999). Thus, the efficacy of PONV prediction models is affected by ethnic differences.

In the previous section, risk factors of PONV are listed, which has shown the direction for the construction of PONV prediction models. Numbers of risk factors are closely related to the risk levels; therefore, prediction models can calculate the risk with the number of risk factors.

A study by Mao and Gu (2012) included a total of 1443 anesthetized patients, in which the incidence of postoperative nausea and vomiting was 23.9%. The incidence of PONV in patients undergoing gynecologic surgery can be as high as 42.5%. The higher the postoperative pain classification, the higher the incidence of POV, and the incidence of PONV in patients with severe pain is 32.3%. logistic regression analysis found that women, history of PONV or motion sickness, and general anesthesia are risk factors for PONV, and dexamethasone and haloperidol have anti-PONV effects. The model constructed according to these five relevant factors is $P = 1/1 + eY = -\ 1.158 + 1.051$ (gender) + 0.984

(general anesthesia) + 0.420 (history) − 0.732 (dexamethasone) − 2.050 (haloperidol) [gender: male-0, female = 1; general anesthesia: no = 0, yes = 11; history: no0, yes = 1; dexamethasone: no-0, yes = 1; fluprednisol: no-0, yes = 1]. The area under the curve of the prediction model was 0.705 (95% confidence interval 0.673–0.737). They concluded that women, history of PONV or motion sickness, and general anesthesia are risk factors for PONV in patients, while giving dexamethasone or haloperidol can reduce the risk of PONV occurrence, and the prediction model constructed by logistic regression analysis can be used to assess the probability of PONV in anesthesia patients, thus providing clinical information for the prevention and treatment of PONV in China.

A study by Ji et al. (2021) developed a prediction model for PONV in neurosurgery patients. The formula for the calculation of risk factors for postoperative nausea and vomiting in neurosurgery: Logit $(P) = -2.372 + 0.623 \times$ female + $0.733 \times$ previous history of postoperative nausea and vomiting + $0.898 \times$ history of upper gastrointestinal tract disease + $1.483 \times$ intraoperative blood transfusion + $0.921 \times$ craniotomy. The area under the ROC curve was 0.716, sensitivity 0.750, specificity 0.577, accuracy 0.266, and maximum Yordon index 0.327. The prediction model was tested using the Hosmer-Lemeshow test with $\chi 2 = 8.343$, $P = 0.303$. The fit was good. The results of this study showed that females with, previous history of postoperative nausea and vomiting, history of upper gastrointestinal tract disease, intraoperative blood transfusion, and craniotomy were independent risk factors for postoperative nausea and vomiting in neurosurgery, and the prediction model of postoperative nausea and vomiting based on the above-influencing factors had a better predictive effect and could complete the assessment of the risk of postoperative nausea and vomiting occurrence during the first evaluation of patients admitted to ICU care after surgery. In this study, we combined the comprehensive factors of postoperative nausea and vomiting in neurosurgery and constructed a prediction model to fully assess the potential risk, which is more conducive to early warning identification of patients with postoperative nausea and vomiting in neurosurgery in clinical practice and to reduce the occurrence of related adverse events. The results of the study showed that the model has ideal specificity, sensitivity, and accuracy, with a maximum Yordon index of 0.327 and an area under the curve of 0.716. The model can be used to predict the probability of postoperative nausea and vomiting, to include neurosurgical patients at high risk in the key population for close observation, and to alert physicians for therapeutic interventions if necessary, so as to reduce the occurrence of adverse events caused by postoperative nausea and vomiting, thus achieving Early warning judgment.

During the care-as-usual period, 1022 patients were enrolled, and 458 patients were included during the intervention period in Kappen et al.'s study (Kappen et al. 2015). There was no significant difference in mean predicted PONV risks between allocation periods. PONV risk categories were, however, distributed differently across allocation periods. Several predictor variables have varying baselines, which is likely to explain small differences in the predicted PONV risk distribution.

The intervention on group completed 75%, the care-as-usual group 83% of the follow-up measurements on PONV, and 92% of all patients completed a follow-up measurement (intervention period 87%; care-as-usual period 94%). The intervention period had a PONV incidence of 42%, while the care-as-usual period had a PONV incidence of 50%. In the intervention period, the incidence of PONV was significantly reduced compared to the care-as-usual period (OR: 0.60, 95% confidence interval: 0.43–0.83), and the reduction was greater for high-risk patients (OR interaction term: 0.45, 95% confidence interval: 0.28–0.72). Statistical significance and the number needed to treat (NNT) for the risk-dependent reduction in PONV can be seen in Fig. 1a. Confounder correction using all predictors from the prediction model can explain differences in ORs for the variable predicted risk between complete case analysis and multiple imputations.

Every patient received prophylactic anti-emetics. Sixty-six percent of anesthetists administered prophylactic anti-emetics in accordance with the recommendations from the clinical decision support tool during the intervention period. Care-as-usual compliance increased by 46% after the fictional compliance (the prescription behavior that would have been advised if the decision rule had been active) reached 20%. When compared with the care-as-usual period, 76% of prophylactic anti-emetics were administered appropriately during the anesthesia case during the intervention period. Both the post-anesthesia care unit and the ward did not correlate the timing of prophylactic anti-emetics with PONV. After multiple imputations and confounder adjustments, the linear regression analysis confirmed the increase in prophylactic anti-emetics. As a result of the intervention, anesthesiologists administered more anti-emetic prophylaxis according to risk. The anesthetists administered 0.49 (95% CI: 0.41–0.58) additional anti-emetics for every additional anti-emetic advised during this period.

Kappen et al. evaluated the effects of risk-dependent PONV prophylaxis based on a prediction model's prediction of PONV risks. Using a directive approach, the model presented predicted risks along with treatment recommendations directly to anesthetists in the operating theater. In addition to reducing incidence of PONV within 24 h after surgery, this directive approach clearly increased the administration of risk-dependent anti-emetic prophylaxis to patients.

This study contradicts the outcomes of Kappen et al.'s previous study. An assistive approach was tested in the previous study, which presented only the risk of PONV without recommending therapies. Assistive strategies had little impact on PONV incidence, whereas directive strategies significantly reduced PONV incidence within 24 h (OR: 0.60, 95% CI: 0.43–0.83). As the results of the two studies differ, an actionable recommendation may have a greater impact on clinical practice when accompanied by a prediction model.

Physician behavior was positively affected in this study, as it has been in other PONV decision support studies. A directive decision support tool implemented by Kooij and colleagues resulted in an absolute increase of 40% in compliance, which matches Kappen et al.'s (46%). As in our previous (assistive) study, Frenzel and colleagues (Frenzel et al. 2020) achieved an absolute increase of 5% in compliance by applying an assistive approach. Our directive approach reduced overall absolute risk by 8%, which is in line with other studies that reported similar reductions ranging from 8% to 35%. It is unfortunate that such a comparison lacks value, due to differences in PONV prophylaxis administration, study design, and analysis. In most other studies, there was no randomization, no adjustment for confounding, or no control group. Thus, comparing our results with theirs is difficult.

The directive approach may result in a significant reduction in PONV incidence, but its actual impact on PONV occurrence seems moderate at best and does not even approach its desired result-a "PONV-free hospital." In spite of this, we should not discard risk-dependent strategies for PONV prophylaxis since the actual impact differs from the potential impact. Prior to coming to a conclusion, we need to consider several interactions between clinicians and the decision support tool.

Predictive performance of the prediction model may have been inadequate to improve clinical decision-making. Compared with other PONV prediction models, our prediction model performed well (c-statistic ~0.70). Model-based decisions may not have been superior to clinical judgement with moderate predictive performance. A second factor that may have affected compliance with the recommendations is the interface of the decision support tool. Due to prophylactic anti-emetics being administered either at the beginning or toward the end of an anesthetic case, desensitization may have occurred. The third finding is that physicians did not fully comply with the therapeutic and risk recommendations despite a sizeable increase in risk-dependent PONV prophylaxis. A patient in the highest risk category was advised to take three prophylactic anti-emetics, but only received two of them on average. A number of barriers have been identified in the literature that could contribute to the anesthetists' limited compliance with prediction models and decision support. Fourthly, prophylactic anti-emetics may have become more prevalent because of an overall increase in attention to PONV, not because of the intervention itself. Therefore, decision support systems are sometimes referred to as "reminder systems" since they are designed to increase understanding of a particular patient problem. Prediction models are used as decision support to improve risk-dependent decision-making by using predictions as inputs. Rather than a Hawthorne effect, the decision support tool likely provided information that assisted them in making decisions, as both primary and secondary outcomes resulted in a risk-dependent prediction model.

3 Conclusion

Risk-dependent PONV prevention is efficacious in both clinical trials and clinical practice when a real-time, computer-based prediction model is applied together with risk-based recommendations on PONV prevention. Implementing a risk prediction model in combination with treatment recommendations for each predicted risk can generate better results for clinical decision-making and patient outcomes than applying a prediction model without considering such treatment recommendations. In light of the remaining high resulting incidence of PONV, more liberal use of prophylactic anti-emetics and lower risk thresholds for actionable recommendations may be required to realize a real "PONV-free hospital."

References

Acar HV. Acupuncture and related techniques during perioperative period: a literature review. Complement Ther Med. 2016;29:48–55. https://doi.org/10.1016/j.ctim.2016.09.013. Epub 2016 Sep 13.

Apfel CC, Läärä E, Koivuranta M, Greim CA, Roewer N. A simplified risk score for predicting postoperative nausea and vomiting: conclusions from cross-validations between two centers. Anesthesiology. 1999;91(3):693–700. https://doi.org/10.1097/00000542-199909000-00022.

Apfel CC, Heidrich FM, Jukar-Rao S, Jalota L, Hornuss C, Whelan RP, Zhang K, Cakmakkaya OS. Evidence-based analysis of risk factors for postoperative nausea and vomiting. Br J Anaesth. 2012;109(5):742–53. https://doi.org/10.1093/bja/aes276. Epub 2012 Oct 3.

Athavale A, Athavale T, Roberts DM. Antiemetic drugs: what to prescribe and when. Aust Prescr. 2020;43(2):49–56. https://doi.org/10.18773/austprescr.2020.011. Epub 2020 Apr 1.

Echeverria-Villalobos M, Fiorda-Diaz J, Uribe A, Bergese SD. Postoperative nausea and vomiting in female patients undergoing breast and gynecological surgery: a narrative review of risk factors and prophylaxis. Front Med (Lausanne). 2022;9:909982. https://doi.org/10.3389/fmed.2022.909982.

Elvir-Lazo OL, White PF, Yumul R, Cruz EH. Management strategies for the treatment and prevention of postoperative/postdischarge nausea and vomiting: an updated review. F1000Res. 2020;9:F1000 Faculty Rev-983. https://doi.org/10.12688/f1000research.21832.1.

Frenzel F, Hollaender S, Fries P, Stroeder R, Stroeder J. Jejunal obstruction due to rare internal hernia between skeletonized external iliac artery and vein as late complication of laparoscopic hysterectomy with pelvic lymphadenectomy-case report and review of literature. Arch Gynecol Obstet. 2020;302(5):1075–80. https://doi.org/10.1007/s00404-020-05724-x. Epub 2020 Aug 7.

Gan TJ, Diemunsch P, Habib AS, Kovac A, Kranke P, Meyer TA, Watcha M, Chung F, Angus S, Apfel CC, Bergese SD, Candiotti KA, Chan MT, Davis PJ, Hooper VD, Lagoo-Deenadayalan S, Myles P, Nezat G, Philip BK, Tramèr MR. Society for ambulatory anesthesia. Consensus guidelines for the management of postoperative nausea and vomiting. Anesth Analg. 2014;118(1):85–113. https://doi.org/10.1213/ANE.0000000000000002. Erratum in: Anesth Analg. 2014; 118(3): 689. Erratum in: Anesth Analg. 2015 Feb; 120(2): 494.

Haber SL, Graybill A, Minasian A. Amisulpride: a new drug for management of postoperative nausea and vomiting. Ann Pharmacother. 2021;55(10):1276–82. https://doi.org/10.1177/1060028020987012. Epub 2021 Jan 8.

Horn CC, Wallisch WJ, Homanics GE, Williams JP. Pathophysiological and neurochemical mechanisms of postoperative nausea and vomiting. Eur J Pharmacol. 2014;722:55–66. https://doi.org/10.1016/j.ejphar.2013.10.037. Epub 2013 Oct 26.

Ji L, Li XY, Zhang L, Qian XY, Li J. Construction and evaluation of a predictive model for postoperative nausea and vomiting in neurosurgery. J Nurs. 2021;36(10):35–7.

Kappen TH, Vergouwe Y, van Wolfswinkel L, Kalkman CJ, Moons KG, van Klei WA. Impact of adding therapeutic recommendations to risk assessments from a prediction model for postoperative nausea and vomiting. Br J Anaesth. 2015;114(2):252–60. https://doi.org/10.1093/bja/aeu321. Epub 2014 Oct 1.

Koivuranta M, Läärä E, Snåre L, Alahuhta S. A survey of postoperative nausea and vomiting. Anaesthesia. 1997;52:443–9.

Kovac AL. Postoperative nausea and vomiting in pediatric patients. Paediatr Drugs. 2021;23(1):11–37. https://doi.org/10.1007/s40272-020-00424-0. Epub 2020 Oct 27.

Law MR, Wald NJ, Morris JK, Jordan RE. Value of low dose combination treatment with blood pressure lowering drugs: analysis of 354 randomised trials. BMJ. 2003;326(7404):1427. https://doi.org/10.1136/bmj.326.7404.1427.

Mao Y, Gu EW. Analysis of influencing factors of postoperative nausea and vomiting and construction of prediction model[C]. The 2nd global Chinese anesthesia conference 5th National Academic Forum for young anesthesiologists of the year 2012; 2012. p. 160–1.

Mawe GM, Hoffman JM. Serotonin signalling in the gut-functions, dysfunctions and therapeutic targets. Nat Rev Gastroenterol Hepatol. 2013;10(8):473–86. https://doi.org/10.1038/nrgastro.2013.105. Epub 2013 Jun 25. Erratum in: Nat Rev Gastroenterol Hepatol. 2013; 10(10): 564.

Ngo AL, Orhurhu V, Urits I, Delfin EO, Sharma M, Jones MR, Viswanath O, Urman RD. Extended release granisetron: review of pharmacologic considerations and clinical role in the perioperative setting. Saudi J Anaesth. 2019;13(3):231–6. https://doi.org/10.4103/sja.SJA_817_18.

Shaikh SI, Nagarekha D, Hegade G, Marutheesh M. Postoperative nausea and vomiting: a simple yet complex problem. Anesth Essays Res. 2016;10(3):388–96. https://doi.org/10.4103/0259-1162.179310.

Theriot J, Wermuth HR, Ashurst JV. Antiemetic Serotonin-5-HT3 receptor blockers. In: StatPearls. Treasure Island (FL): StatPearls Publishing; 2022. https://www.ncbi.nlm.nih.gov/books/NBK513318/.

van den Bosch JE, Kalkman CJ, Vergouwe Y, Van Klei WA, Bonsel GJ, Grobbee DE, Moons KG. Assessing the applicability of scoring systems for predicting postoperative nausea and vomiting. Anaesthesia. 2005;60(4):323–31. https://doi.org/10.1111/j.1365-2044.2005.04121.x.

Veiga-Gil L, Pueyo J, López-Olaondo L. Postoperative nausea and vomiting: physiopathology, risk factors, prophylaxis and treatment. Rev Esp Anestesiol Reanim. 2017;64(4):223–32. https://doi.org/10.1016/j.redar.2016.10.001. Epub 2016 Dec 29. English, Spanish.

Yoo JH, Kim SI, Chung JW, Jun MR, Han YM, Kim YJ. Aprepitant in combination with palonosetron for the prevention of postoperative nausea and vomiting in female patients using intravenous patient-controlled analgesia. Korean J Anesthesiol. 2018;71(6):440–6. https://doi.org/10.4097/kja.d.18.00011. Epub 2018 May 30.

Artificial Intelligence in Pain Management

Bifa Fan

Pain management has always been one of the core topics discussed in anesthesiology. The realm of pain management that benefits from AI may penetrate every stage of anesthesia and surgery such as the prediction of opioid prescription, and more importantly, the diagnosis of pain. The identification of pain was difficult even with the assistance of imaging techniques, not to mention diagnosing pain by the widely used various scales. Fortunately, researchers have developed various models and methods based on machine learning to identify pain in a more objective and scientific manner. Besides, opioids play a critical role in acute or chronic postoperative pain management. Yet, considering the addictive nature of opioid therapies and their side effects, patients who suffer from postoperative pain may better be discriminated to get individualized therapies. There are studies exploring the potential of machine learning methods to achieve the goal of personalizing patients' pain treatment.

B. Fan (✉)
Department of Pain Medicine, China-Japan Friendship Hospital, Beijing, China

1 AI in Chronic Pain Diagnosis and Care

Automated detection of pain is a topic of great interest in the healthcare field because pain is not only an important indicator for medical diagnosis but also a barrier that affects patient recovery in the intensive care unit and after surgery (Joshi and Ogunnaike 2005). The study of Anderson et al. showed that accurate pain assessment plays a key role in precise pain control (Anderson et al. 2000). Currently, pain assessment is usually performed by a professional nurse through a verbal examination, which is referred to as self-report. However, such a way of assessment is not always completed successfully due to factors such as the patient's age, specific medical conditions, or language barriers. In addition, pain is a subjective sensation and the way it is described varies across cultures. Consequently, if the automatic and scientific assessment of pain can be addressed by AI, it will greatly improve the efficiency of pain diagnosis and treatment outcomes.

Researchers have been marching toward the goal of AI diagnosis of pain. Typically, facial action units (AUs) have been used to encode facial motion corresponding to different facial expressions, including pain. As manifested by Rudovic et al. (2015), the task of AU intensity estimation is very challenging due to the high variability of facial expressions depending on the environment, such as illumination, head

M. Xia, H. Jiang (eds.), *Artificial Intelligence in Anesthesiology*,
https://doi.org/10.1007/978-981-99-5925-9_9

movements, or expressions of specific objects. As a complex task, AU intensity estimation has gained much attention in the last two decades for general facial motion analysis. Whereas, the study of Rodriguez et al. used the raw facial image as the input of the convolutional neural network (CNN) instead of facial markers, which is different from previous studies. They confronted the binary pain recognition task for facial images from a deep learning perspective, achieving state-of-the-art results in comparison to the leave-one-subject setting (Rodriguez et al. 2022). Thus, this exposed the problem of deciding which method was more persuasive when other works have substaintiated their results with details such as accuracy, area under the curve (AUC), subject exclusion, and non-exclusion settings. They considered subject exclusion to be crucial and therefore provided all results computed in this manner. They announced that their method of training deep CNNs for pain level estimation has provided good results, and they have shown that using RNNs to exploit the temporal relationship between frames can improve the results. By training a CNN end to end for pain level estimation, their method obtained an AUC of 89.6, which increased to 93.3 when the same CNN was used to extract features to train a RNN. In addition, they demonstrated the generality of their method by obtaining an accuracy of 97.2% on the Extended Cohn-Kanade (CK+) facial emotion recognition dataset, compared to the state-of-the-art method. The result they achieved was a competitive score compared to the most advanced methods (97.3%) (Zhao et al. 2016).

Pain identification is not limited to imaging techniques; Ben-Israel et al. developed a nociceptive level (NOL) index that was based on a machine learning analysis of photoreceptor maps and skin conduction waveforms recorded in 25 patients undergoing elective surgery (Ben-Israel et al. 2013). However, the NOL index was based on a target described as a composite index of stimulation and analgesia that was defined and validated in the same study, embracing an arbitrary ranking of intraoperative toxic stimuli. Gram et al. used machine learning to analyze the EEG signals of 81 patients trying to predict patients who responded to opioid therapy for acute pain; the results showed that the preoperative EEG assessment was only 65% accurate for patients who responded to postoperative opioid therapy (Gram et al. 2017). In addition, Olesen et al. conducted a large data study looking for single nucleotide polymorphisms in 1237 cancer patients that could predict opioid dose in these patients; however, their study did not find any association of single nucleotide polymorphisms with opioid dose in this population (Olesen et al. 2018).

Chronic pain is a complex condition that is often misdiagnosed because it shares symptoms with other syndromes. In this context, several studies have proposed different machine learning algorithms to classify or predict chronic pain conditions. These algorithms employ a variety of data types, ranging from questionnaire-based self-reported data to state-of-the-art brain imaging techniques. In Santana et al.'s study, they evaluated the sensitivity of different algorithms and datasets for the classification of chronic pain syndromes (Santana et al. 2020). Along with the evaluation, they highlighted important methodological steps that should be considered when conducting machine learning experiments. The best results were obtained with the ensemble-based algorithm and the dataset containing the maximum information diversity, resulting in an area under the receiver operating curve value of approximately 0.85. In addition, the performance of the algorithm is closely related to the hyper-parameters. Therefore, a good hyper-parameter optimization strategy should be used to extract the most information from the algorithm. These findings supported the idea that machine learning can be a powerful tool for a better understanding of chronic pain conditions.

Specifically, researchers have achieved progress in predicting chronic pain disease with machine learning. For example, Wang et al. dig deep into the prediction of postherpetic neuralgia in patients with herpes zoster by machine learning (Wang et al. 2020). They intended to develop a predictive model to evaluate whether patients with shingles would develop PHN. They reviewed 52 patients with shingles and classified them according to whether they had PHN. Risk factors associated with PHN were identified by univariate analysis. Machine learning using logistic regression and random forest algorithms was completed, and then the prediction accuracies of the two algorithms were compared to select the superior algorithm to predict the next 60 new cases. The results showed that age, NRS score, rash site, Charlson comorbidity index (CCI) score, antiviral therapy, and immunosuppression were all associated with the development of PHN. The NRS score was the most strongly associated factor with a significance of 0.31. As for accuracy, random forest had an accuracy of 96.24%, which was superior to logistic regression's 92.83%. Then, the random forest model was used to predict 60 newly diagnosed herpes zoster patients with an accuracy of 88.33% and a 95% confidence interval (CI) of 77.43–95.18%.

Furthermore, experts developed and examined the efficacy of AI in improving the treatment strategy for chronic pain. Cognitive behavioral therapy for chronic pain (CBT-CP) is a safe and effective alternative to opioid analgesics. Piette et al. applied the principles of "reinforcement learning" (a field of artificial intelligence) to develop an evidence-based, personalized CBT pain management service that automatically adapts to the unique and changing needs of each patient (AI-CBT). AI-CBT uses feedback from patients about their pain-related functional progress, measured daily through pedometer steps, to automatically personalize the intensity and type (Piette et al. 2016). In their later research, they made a comparison between AI-CBT-CP personalized patient treatment and standard telephone CBT-CP treatment. The results showed that among 278 participants, the 3-month mean RMDQ score difference between AI-CBT-CP and standard CBT-CP was −0.72 points (95% CI, −2.06 to 0.62) and the 6-month difference was −1.24 points (95% CI, −2.48 to 0); no inferiority criterion was met at both the 3- and 6-month end points ($P < 0.001$ for both). Over half of the participants receiving AI-CBT-CP had clinically meaningful improvements at 6 months as indicated by RMDQ (37% vs 19%; $P = 0.01$) and pain intensity scores (29% vs 17%; $P = 0.03$) (Piette et al. 2022).

2 AI in Intraoperative Pain Management

When it comes to intraoperative pain management, quantifying the patient's NOL and adjusting the analgesic drug infusion during anesthesia have still been a challenge. Consequently, applying machine learning techniques to assist clinicians with analgesic drug administration are considered to improve pain management quality during anesthesia. As done by Gonzalez-Cava et al. (2020), they evaluated the Analgesia Nociception Index (ANI) as a guiding variable for opioid infusion rate regulation. The ANI monitor—Physiodoloris performed heart rate variability (HRV) analysis to measure the effect of respiratory sinus arrhythmia (RSA). The ANI values together with hemodynamic information were superior to non-specific conventional signs such as heart rate and blood pressure to quantify NOL and can predict dose changes to prevent hemodynamic events before they occur (Gonzalez-Cava et al. 2020). The efficiency of the support vector machine (SVM) classifier using ANI as a guidance variable can be demonstrated with an accuracy of 86.21% (83.62–87.93%), a precision of 86.11% (83.78–88.57%), a recall of 91.18% (88.24–91.18%), a specificity of 79.17% (75–83.33%), an AUC of 0.89 (0.87–0.90) and a kappa index of 0.71 (0.66–0.75) (Gonzalez-Cava et al. 2020).

Likewise, Tighe et al. (2012) conducted a study of artificial intelligence and intraoperative pain management, aiming to determine if a machine learning classifier could predict which patients would require preoperative acute pain service (APS) consultation. They reviewed the records of 9860 surgical patients between January 1 and June 30, 2010. Surgical cases requiring preoperative acute pain service consultation were classified and compared based on the ability or inability of the machine learning classifier. The classifiers were then optimized using ensemble techniques. Computational efficiency was measured by the central processor processing time required for model training. The classifier was tested using the full feature set, as well as a reduced feature set optimized using a merit-based dimensionality reduction strategy. The machine learning classifier correctly predicted 92.3% (95% confidence interval [CI], 91.8–92.8) of requests for preoperative acute pain service consultations across all surgical cases. The Bayesian approach yielded the highest area under the receiver operating curve (0.87, 95% CI 0.84–0.89) and the shortest training time (0.0018 s, 95% CI, 0.0017–0.0019 for the naïve Bayes Updateable algorithm). The combination of a high-performance machine learning classifier did not yield a higher area under the receiver operating curve than its component classifiers. The dimensionality reduction decreased the computational requirements of multiple classifiers but did not adversely affect classification performance.

3 AI in Postoperative Pain Management

In the field of pain medicine, artificial intelligence is emerging as a competent helper. Its powerful and sophisticated analytical capabilities make a better understanding of the pathophysiology of pain become possible. Gonzalez-Cava et al. used machine learning to analyze differences in functional magnetic resonance imaging (MRI) data collected from human volunteers who were exposed to painful and non-painful thermal stimuli (Gonzalez-Cava et al. 2017). They illustrated that machine learning analysis of whole brain scans was more successful in accurately identifying pain than traditional analysis of individual brain regions associated with nociception. In addition, good results have been achieved with respect to postoperative pain, probably considering the complexity of the variables that contribute to the development of postoperative pain, both in terms of their numbers and relationships (Gonzalez-Cava et al. 2017). Barry et al. in their analysis of factors associated with rebound pain after peripheral nerve block, found that compared to other analysis methods, especially with multivariate logistic regression models, machine learning techniques, especially the "logistic model tree attribute selection classifier," was able to uncover new variables not previously considered and proved to have the best performance (Barry et al. 2021). Parthipan et al., on the other hand, used machine learning techniques to better understand the relationship between postoperative pain and depression (Parthipan et al. 2019). They concluded that thanks to the use of these new analytical techniques, the first groundbreaking demonstration of the known ability of selective 5-hydroxytryptamine reuptake inhibitors (SSRIs) to suppress the potency of prodrug opioids had an impact on worse pain control. Machine learning has proven useful not only in pain risk prediction but also in supporting clinical decision-making in acute pain services (APS) (Tighe et al. 2012).

Opioids play a crucial role in acute postoperative pain management. Nair et al. conducted a study on machine learning approach to predict postoperative opioid requirements in ambulatory surgery patients (Nair et al. 2020). Their goal was to develop machine learning models to predict the postoperative opioid requirements of patients undergoing ambulatory surgery. To develop these models, they used a perioperative dataset that included 13,700 patients (18 years of age and older) who underwent outpatient surgery from 2016 to 2018. These data, which included patient, procedure, and provider factors that may influence postoperative pain and opioid requirements, were randomly divided into training (80%) and validation (20%) datasets. Different classes of machine learning models were developed using the training dataset to predict categorical levels of postoperative opioid need and then evaluated on the validation dataset. Prediction accuracy was used to differentiate the performance of the models. The accuracy of the five classes of models developed was as follows at two different stages of surgery: (1) pre-surgery—Multinomial Logistic Regression: 71%, Naive Bayes: 67%, Neural Network: 30%, Random Forest: 72%, Extreme Gradient Boost: 71%; (2) End of surgery—Multinomial Logistic Regression: 71%, Naive Bayes: 63%, Neural Network: 32%,

Random Forest: 72%, Extreme Gradient Boost: 70%. Analysis of the sensitivity of the best-performing Random Forest model showed higher prediction accuracy for lower opioid demand (89%) compared to higher opioid demand (43%). The importance of features (relative importance percentage) predicted by the model showed that type of surgery (15.4%), medical history (12.9%), and time of surgery (12.0%) were the three features that contributed the most to the model predictions. Overall, patient and procedure features contributed 65% and 35% to model predictions, respectively. Machine learning models can be used to predict postoperative opioid requirements for ambulatory surgery patients and potentially help better manage their acute postoperative pain.

Similarly, another research performed by Lu et al. focused on the development and verification of a machine learning algorithm that can predict patients at risk for delayed postoperative opioid use after receiving elective knee arthroscopy (Lu et al. 2022). They reviewed the data at a tertiary academic medical center and identified adult patients undergoing knee arthroscopy between 2016 and 2018. They defined prolonged postoperative opioid consumption as opioid consumption lasting for at least 150 days after surgery. Five machine learning algorithms were evaluated for their ability to predict the prolonged opioid consumption outcome. The assessment tools included discrimination, calibration, and decision curve analysis. Overall, 60 (20.3%) of the 381 patients included showed continued opioid consumption postoperatively. The factors determined for the prediction of prolonged postoperative opioid prescription were reduced preoperative scores for the following patient-reported results: the IKDC, KOOS ADL, VR12 MCS, KOOS pain, and KOOS Sport and Activities. The ensemble model achieved the best performance based on discrimination (AUC = 0.74), calibration, and decision curve analysis. This model was integrated into a web-based open-access application capable of providing prediction and interpretation. With appropriate external validation, the algorithm currently developed enhances the timely identification of patients at risk for long-term opioid use. Reduced scores on preoperative patient-reported outcomes, symptom duration, and perioperative oral morphine equivalents were identified as novel predictors of prolonged postoperative opioid use. The predictive model can be easily deployed in a clinical setting to identify patients at risk, thus allowing providers to optimize modifiable risk factors and counsel patients appropriately preoperatively.

Apart from being used as a tool to diagnose pain, NOL also imposes positive impacts on guiding the use of opioids in managing postoperative pain. Meijer et al. found that the majority of postoperative patients reported moderate to severe pain and that pain may be associated with under- or over-dosing of opioids during surgery (Meijer et al. 2020). Objective guidance on opioid dosing using the NOL index could help improve postoperative pain control in patients. Specifically, the NOL index is a multiparametric artificial intelligence-driven index designed to monitor nociception during surgery, potentially leading to more appropriate analgesic protocols and better surgical outcomes. They tested whether NOL-guided opioid dosage during general anesthesia reduced postoperative pain. In this two-center RCT study, 50 patients undergoing abdominal surgery under fentanyl/sevoflurane anesthesia were randomly assigned to either the NOL-guided fentanyl dose group or the standard of care group, in which fentanyl dosage was determined hemodynamically. Patients' postoperative pain levels were assessed in the PACU. Results showed a median postoperative pain score of 3.2 (interquartile range 1.3–4.3) and 4.8 (3.0–5.3) in the NOL-guided and standard care groups, respectively ($P = 0.006$). Postoperative morphine consumption (standard deviation) was 0.06 (0.07) mg/kg (NOL-guided group) and 0.09 (0.09) mg/kg (control group; $P = 0.204$). During surgery, the dose of fentanyl did not differ between groups (NOL-guided group: 6.4 [4.2] μg/kg vs. standard care: 6.0 [2.2] μg/kg, $P = 0.749$), although the difference between patients in the NOL-guided group was greater (coefficient of variation: 66% in the NOL-guided group and 37% in the standard care group). This suggests some improvement in postoperative pain scores (1.6 points) in patients under NOL guidance, although there was no difference in intraoperative and postoperative fentanyl and morphine consumption.

References

Anderson KO, et al. Minority cancer patients and their providers: pain management attitudes and practice. Cancer. 2000;88(8):1929–38.

Barry GS, Bailey JG, Sardinha J, et al. Factors associated with rebound pain after peripheral nerve block for ambulatory surgery. Br J Anaesth. 2021;126:862–71.

Ben-Israel N, Kliger M, Zuckerman G, Katz Y, Edry R. Monitoring the nociception level: a multi-parameter approach. J Clin Monit Comput. 2013;27:659–68.

Gonzalez-Cava JM, Arnay R, Perez JAM, Leon A, Martin M, Jove-Perez E, Calvo-Rolle JL, CasteleiroRoca JL, Juez FJD, Garcia HP, AlfonsoCendon J, Gonzalez LS, Quintian H, Corchado E. A machine learning based system for analgesic drug delivery. In: International joint conference SOCO'17-CISIS'17-ICEUTE'17, vol. 649; 2017. p. 461–70.

Gonzalez-Cava JM, Arnay R, León A, et al. Machine learning based method for the evaluation of the analgesia nociception index in the assessment of general anesthesia. Comput Biol Med. 2020;118:103645.

Gram M, Erlenwein J, Petzke F, Falla D, Przemeck M, Emons MI, Reuster M, Olesen SS, Drewes AM. Prediction of postoperative opioid analgesia using clinical-experimental parameters and electroencephalography. Eur J Pain. 2017;21:264–77.

Joshi GP, Ogunnaike BO. Consequences of inadequate postoperative pain relief and chronic persistent postoperative pain. Anesthesiol Clin North Am. 2005;23(1):21–36.

Lu Y, Forlenza E, Wilbur RR, Lavoie-Gagne O, Fu MC, Yanke AB, Cole BJ, Verma N, Forsythe B. Machine-learning model successfully predicts patients at risk for prolonged postoperative opioid use following elective knee arthroscopy. Knee Surg Sports Traumatol Arthrosc. 2022;30(3):762–72. https://doi.org/10.1007/s00167-020-06421-7. Epub 2021 Jan 9.

Meijer F, Honing M, Roor T, Toet S, Calis P, Olofsen E, Martini C, van Velzen M, Aarts L, Niesters M, Boon M, Dahan A. Reduced postoperative pain using nociception level-guided fentanyl dosing during sevoflurane anaesthesia: a randomised controlled trial. Br J Anaesth. 2020;125(6):1070–8. https://doi.org/10.1016/j.bja.2020.07.057. Epub 2020 Sep 17.

Nair AA, Velagapudi MA, Lang JA, Behara L, Venigandla R, Velagapudi N, et al. Machine learning approach to predict postoperative opioid requirements in ambulatory surgery patients. PLoS One. 2020;15(7):e0236833. https://doi.org/10.1371/journal.pone.0236833.

Olesen AE, Grønlund D, Gram M, Skorpen F, Drewes AM, Klepstad P. Prediction of opioid dose in cancer pain patients using genetic profiling: not yet an option with support vector machine learning. BMC Res Notes. 2018;11:78.

Parthipan A, Banerjee I, Humphreys K, et al. Predicting inadequate postoperative pain management in depressed patients: a machine learning approach. PLoS One. 2019;14:e0210575.

Piette JD, Krein SL, Striplin D, Marinec N, Kerns RD, Farris KB, Singh S, An L, Heapy AA. Patient-centered pain care using artificial intelligence and mobile health tools: protocol for a randomized study funded by the US department of veterans affairs health services research and development program. JMIR Res Protoc. 2016;5(2):e53. https://doi.org/10.2196/resprot.4995.

Piette JD, Newman S, Krein SL, Marinec N, Chen J, Williams DA, Edmond SN, Driscoll M, LaChappelle KM, Kerns RD, Maly M, Kim HM, Farris KB, Higgins DM, Buta E, Heapy AA. Patient-centered pain care using artificial intelligence and Mobile health tools: a randomized comparative effectiveness trial. JAMA Intern Med. 2022;182(9):975–83. https://doi.org/10.1001/jamainternmed.2022.3178.

Rodriguez P, Cucurull G, Gonzalez J, Gonfaus JM, Nasrollahi K, Moeslund TB, Roca FX. Deep pain: exploiting long short-term memory networks for facial expression classification. IEEE Trans Cybern. 2022;52(5):3314–24. https://doi.org/10.1109/TCYB.2017.2662199. Epub 2022 May 19.

Rudovic O, Pavlovic V, Pantic M. Context-sensitive dynamic ordinal regression for intensity estimation of facial action units. IEEE Trans Pattern Anal Mach Intell. 2015;37(5):944–58.

Santana AN, de Santana CN, Montoya P. Chronic pain diagnosis using machine learning, questionnaires, and QST: a sensitivity experiment. Diagnostics (Basel). 2020;10(11):958. https://doi.org/10.3390/diagnostics10110958.

Tighe PJ, Lucas SD, Edwards DA, et al. Use of machine-learning classifiers to predict requests for preoperative acute pain service consultation. Pain Med. 2012;13:1347–57.

Wang XX, Zhang Y, Fan BF. Predicting postherpetic neuralgia in patients with herpes zoster by machine learning: a retrospective study. Pain Ther. 2020;9(2):627–35. https://doi.org/10.1007/s40122-020-00196-y. Epub 2020 Sep 11.

Zhao X, et al. Peak-piloted deep network for facial expression recognition. In: Proc. Eur. Conf. Comput. Vis. Amsterdam, the Netherlands; 2016. p. 425–42.

Clinical Decision Support System

Hong Jiang

The anesthesia record is a major component of clinical anesthesia work, and patients' perioperative data is of referential meaning for subsequent anesthesia management. The current anesthesia information management systems (AIMS) used in major hospitals can collect data from sources such as monitors, hospital information systems, ventilators, and anesthesia workstations in real time, while the anesthesiologist records the patient's fluid balance status, surgery, medication, special events, and other information according to the intraoperative anesthesia management condition. All these records form a comprehensive database of real-time patient information during the surgery.

1 Development of Clinical Decision Support System

With the growing popularity of AIMS, researchers have used machine learning to analyze the comprehensive database, and clinical decision support system (CDSS), a hardware system that provides timely decision aids for anesthesiologists and helps to exterminate errors, was then developed. CDSS collects data from the AIMS and categorizes it into usable data by transforming, filtering, and filling in the gaps (Sutton et al. 2020). The decision processor applies algorithms to the usable data and determines whether to notify or alert (e.g., pop-up messages or flashing buttons) on the AIMS according to the set decision rules, and the anesthesiologist makes an autonomous decision about the next step in the treatment plan based on the alert prompts.

In the medical field, the development of computer systems that can use patient data and clinical guidelines to simulate the human decision-making process and accelerate the automation of clinicians' reasoning and judgment has been a topic of debate for decades. As early as 1968, Lusted began researching ways to more accurately implement human workflows in medical practice on computers (Ambinder 2005). However, the development of such systems is a complex process and demands multidisciplinary task that requires the integration of knowledge and decisions from the clinical domain to make the CDSS adaptable to the workflow of the entire healthcare system practice. In recent years, the CONFlexFlow (clinic context-based flexible workFlow) system, a clinical context-based flexible work system, has successfully integrated clinical workflows into CDSS, accelerating the progress of computer-based diagnosis and treatment research (Yao and Kumar 2013). Despite the rapid development of CDSS, there are no systematic conceptual descriptions and implementation methods for CDSS in data mining and

H. Jiang (✉)
Department of Anesthesiology, Shanghai Ninth People's Hospital, Shanghai Jiao Tong University School of Medicine, Shanghai, China

M. Xia, H. Jiang (eds.), *Artificial Intelligence in Anesthesiology*,
https://doi.org/10.1007/978-981-99-5925-9_10

decision-making. Knowledge-based CDSS uses natural language processing techniques to mimic the knowledge and experience of experts and build expert systems to make diagnostic strategies including disease prediction and matching treatment plans (Afzal et al. 2015).

As the complexity of the medical treatment process has escalated in recent years, various medical fields need CDSS to provide various treatment options for clinicians to choose or modify, in addition to strict paradigm clinical decision-making. Machine learning and artificial intelligence breakthroughs have made it easier for CDSS to mine information from large amounts of historical data and be more accurate and relevant in predicting clinical outcomes. Non-knowledge-based CDSS is based on big data to build and train classification models or prediction models, and then perform disease identification diagnosis and risk prediction (Huang et al. 2020). Such CDSS are data mining using various machine learning methods. Arooj et al. used Bayesian networks, support vector machine (SVM), and function tree (FT) as algorithms for heart disease detection assisted decision systems and compared their accuracy; data from the Stanford Cancer Center related database were used to demonstrate the high accuracy and interpretability of the method and to demonstrate a decision support system for personalized treatment of metastatic cancer (Arooj et al. 2022).

2 Adoption of CDSS in the Clinical Context

CDSS may not be fully adopted by end users just because it is available. As a result, even though evidence of CDSS's benefits increases, the adoption rate still remains low (Laka et al. 2021). The adoption rate of CDSS in healthcare organizations is lower than expected, with 96% of alerts or recommendations being ignored or overridden (Chow et al. 2016; Liberati et al. 2017; Moxey et al. 2010) as a result of end users' negative attitudes, evasion, and skepticism, as well as unanticipated effects on clinical workflows (Chung et al. 2017; Kortteisto et al. 2012; Ozkaynak et al. 2018).

An array of interdependent factors influences the success of the implementation of systems like CDSS, including clinical culture, processes, workflows, and professional norms (Kilsdonk et al. 2017). Several factors, including system, organizational, and human factors, contribute to the challenge of implementing CDSS, as Yusof et al. discovered (Yusof et al. 2008). It is difficult to ensure that improving one aspect of the care process does not have unintended consequences in another because of this complexity.

Adopting CDSS can also be challenging due to its scope which goes beyond that of an information technology tool. It integrates a paradigm of evidence-based practice into everyday clinical practice (Sutton et al. 2020). Scientists report that the CDSS can sometimes challenge deep-seated beliefs about professional autonomy and hierarchies of authority in the clinical setting, which can lead to skepticism about its use (Liberati et al. 2017). Studies have examined CDSS adoption based on technical appropriateness and user experience (Camacho et al. 2020; Catho et al. 2020; Jung et al. 2020), but few have examined how end-user characteristics influence perceptions.

2.1 Barriers and Facilitators in the Adoption

2.1.1 External Factors

There was a lack of support and training provided by organizations, which led to a lack of confidence in the system and made it difficult for users to resolve technical problems, thus discouraging CDSS adoption (Lai et al. 2006; Trivedi et al. 2002). The adoption of any new technology is also influenced by cultural factors according to organizational theories (Tsiknakis and Kouroubali 2009). It was found that young clinicians were more prone to obtain organizational support before taking up CDSS for antibiotic management, perhaps due to the profound impact of the clinical hierarchy and seniors' preferences on their practice (Allard 1998) as seniors were less willing to use CDSS.

It is one of the fundamental constructs of UTAUT to make sure the system is easy to use. In the survey, clinicians rated ease of use as one of the most important factors in adopting and adhering to CDSS for antibiotic management. This is in accordance with measures in the information system (IS) success model proposed by DeLone and Mclean which relates user satisfaction and adoption to ease of use (Yusof et al. 2008; DeLone and McLean 2004). Primary care clinicians and those who have used CDSS before also regard ease of use as one of the most significant features of CDSS adoption. Features such as limited consultation time, workload, and the potentially compromised direct communication with patients limited by the time required to navigate the system, make ease of use a highly cherishable requirement for the successful execution of CDSS in primary care (Lugtenberg et al. 2015a, 2015b; Short et al. 2003).

User trust that the system is right for their specific requirements affects system effort expectations and perceived benefit (Lugtenberg et al. 2015a). Clinical experience was associated with a preference for end-user consultation as a facilitator of CDSS implementation by clinicians with longer work experience. Similarly, clinicians with more clinical experience (>11 years) who felt CDSS threatened their clinical autonomy were more likely to see it that way. CDSS may be adopted, trusted, and implemented more effectively if experienced clinicians are included in the development and implementation processes.

2.1.2 Internal Factors

The lack of confidence in the content of the CDSS was frequently reported as the most frequent barrier to the adoption of the CDSS for antibiotic management in our study. CDSS non-users expressed this concern in our study, suggesting that it might be because they do not fully understand how the system gathers information to guide recommendations, they lack trust in the personnel who developed the system, and they do not agree with its content (Khairat et al. 2018; Shibl et al. 2013). Many clinicians are hesitant to engage with CDSS because they fear that it will compromise their clinical judgments (Cabana et al. 1999; Goud et al. 2010). It appears that end-users' reluctance to adopt CDSS may be a result of perceptions about the system rather than actual experience with it since clinicians who have experience related to CDSS are less likely to believe it would compromise their professional autonomy. CDSS is also less likely to be used by experienced clinicians due to their concern that it would compromise established work practices and reduce autonomy over clinical processes and decisions. In the CDSS system, younger clinicians are more confident and have better technological literacy (Laka et al. 2021; Leslie et al. 2006). CDSS users are more likely to be younger clinicians than senior clinicians, as our results support this literature. Clinical engagement with experienced clinicians is essential to overcome barriers to CDSS adoption.

Additionally, end users may be resistant to CDSS adoption for antibiotic management due to clinicians' time constraints and potential workflow disruptions. CDSS uptake and use are negatively impacted by a lack of a fit between relevance and timeliness of recommendations, as shown in previous studies (Moxey et al. 2010; Belard et al. 2016). Furthermore, it was discovered that time and workflow constraints were perceived as more of a barrier to CDSS adoption in primary care. It has been noted that despite workflow disruptions and time constraints (high workloads), CDSS adoption in primary care is limited because clinical data needs to be assessed within a short consultation.

Several moderating factors have a significant impact on clinicians' behavior when it comes to adopting digital health systems, such as age, clinical experience, and digital health literacy. According to the wider literature, these factors are related to users' perception of the usefulness of other digital health systems and their intention to adopt them (Ayaz and Yanartaş 2020; Zuiderwijk et al. 2015; Bandyopadhyay and Barnes 2012). Based on these moderating factors, Jacob et al. suggest that clinicians should understand the users' inclinations and promote a cultural shift among all clinicians to enhance system adoption (Cho et al. 2013). Developing guidelines and policy frameworks for CDSS adoption for antibiotic management should be the focus of future research. We found that these types of CDSS are adopted and used based on a range of individual and setting characteristics. There is a need to address organizational barriers and identify optimal structures to support CDSS implementation in terms of planning, management, leadership, and communication.

2.2 Considerations in the Implementation of CDSS

There is a reasonable case for implementing systems that simulate human decision-making. The ability to automate reasoning and judgment was recognized by researchers decades ago. A better understanding of the human judgment processes involved in diagnosis, for instance, could lead to more accurate computer models of diagnosis (Braun and Clarke 2006).

2.2.1 Does the CDSS Simulate Clinical Assessment with Feedback Loops?

It can be of great value to combine clinician cognition with available clinical information when making clinical decisions. In the literature, several approaches and methods have been discussed for clinical reasoning (Corbin and Strauss 2015). To make a complete and successful differential diagnosis, the physician often requests extra information (e.g., more examinations and radiology tests). The literature has discussed human diagnostic problem solving both domain-independently (Trivedi et al. 2002) as well as the problem of disease diagnosis (Tsiknakis and Kouroubali 2009). By reassessing existing information or by ordering more clinical tests, a physician can "fill in reasoning gaps" during the clinical cognitive process. In making clinical decisions, this loop (clinician's assessment—clinical data—clinician's assessment) is fundamental. Attempts are being made to replicate this possible de facto clinical uncertainty through the feedback loop. By applying reinforcement learning methods to CDSS design approaches, this loop can be simulated (Allard 1998; DeLone and McLean 2004). There is often an inappropriate amount of care given because of the probabilistic nature of health and disease (Lugtenberg et al. 2015a). The design, therefore, needs to take this into account by recognizing, and thereafter evaluating other probable factors, to reduce decision uncertainty. Reinforcement learning methods and dynamic user feedback loop approaches have both been shown to contribute positively to this direction.

2.2.2 Does CDSS Employ Unison Expert Systems and Machine Learning?

By using reasoning approaches, expert systems emulate the cognitive process of making decisions in healthcare settings. As a result of reasoning about knowledge, expert systems solve complex problems using conditional (If-Then-Else) rules. It is difficult to pay attention to all the small, yet non-trivial, clinical details in a clinical setting. A clinical expert system is therefore limited to a defined, very specific domain of decision-making, such as diagnosing a disease. Data-driven machine learning algorithms and traditional knowledge-based systems (mimicking human reasoning using rules) can complement each other well. The purpose of both technologies is to assist clinical decision makers in healthcare settings. Often, the compiled knowledge of a patient does not determine a condition: This is evident when a patient presents in an unexpected or unusual manner or manifests rare symptoms. In order to overcome the aforementioned limitation, the use of enormous historical clinical datasets is suitable, as the datasets are large enough to accommodate patterns of disease for such rare and unique cases. This common objective can be accomplished with greater success when expert systems and machine learning methods are combined with reasoning in decision-making (Khairat et al. 2018).

2.2.3 Does CDSS Use Trends of Physiological Measurements Instead of Cross-Sectional Data?

Physiological measurements and laboratory results are compared to physiological norms when healthcare professionals review patient information (Shibl et al. 2013). By anticipating improved physiological measurements, physicians want to know how patients respond to their therapy of choice rather than just reviewing raw physiological measurements. In addition to assessing the patient's response to the therapy, clinical decision makers consider the physiological values they would expect. When physiologic values for a patient are compared to recent measurements and baselines, treatment effectiveness or progression of the disease can be better understood. Three CDSS design considerations related to this aspect will be elaborated below, namely, inclusion of trends in repeated measures as predictors, modeling the sequence of clinical events, and modeling the temporal distance between clinical events.

It appears that cross-sectional data cannot accurately assess longitudinal care, which may be more important than visit-based indicators (Cabana et al. 1999). Some patients might not be concerned by blood glucose levels of 150 mg/dL if their glucose levels were 180 mg/dL the previous day and 210 mg/dL 2 days ago. While the doctor observed a satisfactory response to therapy despite a 150-mg/dL increase, he did not adjust the therapeutic strategy. Despite this, it would be a different clinical decision for a second patient with a blood glucose measurement of 150 mg/dL if this was the only measurement available. This case would require the physician's attention. It is evident that the model output depends on prior measurements in both scenarios, even though the cross-sectional input value for both of them is the same (blood glucose = 150 mg/dL). A longitudinal medical record is essential to clinical decision support because clinical decisions are longitudinal in nature (Goud et al. 2010). In designing CDSS, it is important to take into consideration temporal trends and fluctuating physiological measurements.

2.2.4 Does CDSS Consider the Temporal Distance of Clinical Events?

In the aforementioned scenario, it is also important to take into account the lag time between diagnoses; that is, how much time passed between diagnosing bacteremia and severe sepsis and septic shock. In order to construct clinically useful events and estimate the severity of those events, the timestamps from EMR data should be used in the analysis. This is especially important to assess the performance of health systems in terms of care delivery and transition and eliminate delays and gaps in service.

3 Problems in the Current Application of CDSS

3.1 Trust Issue of Medical Treatment

When facing diseases such as tumors and cardiovascular diseases, doctors usually inform patients of their current diagnosis. The diagnosis of cancer will disrupt the patients' life state and mental world, and patients will have many concerns to ask doctors and many things on their minds to tell doctors. This requires the doctor to listen to the patient's story, build trust in each other, and deepen mutual understanding in the story, so as to build an emotional foundation for compliance with the diagnosis and treatment later. CDSS, however, changes this traditional diagnostic paradigm. One of the biggest challenges in using CDSS in medicine is the physicians' reluctance to trust and adopt something they do not fully understand, and the lack of trust has slowed progress in the clinical application of these AI tools. In addition to clinician skepticism, patients who lack confidence in AI technology will not be fully convinced.

Most studies have used methods that assess the diagnostic accuracy of deep learning in isolation, an approach that does not fully and truly reflect clinical practice. Many healthcare AI study results are not trusted clinically because the findings do not provide comparisons with diagnoses made by healthcare professionals (physicians) using the same test dataset.

Although CDSS has been systematically learned and continuously trained over a period of time to have a certain basis for clinical application, it cannot be ignored that CDSS still has great limitations in clinical application, both in terms of the level of diagnosis for a single disease and overall thinking about complex diseases, which is actually one of the reasons for the current clinical skepticism about its reliability. Furthermore, the core algorithm and training logic and even the different perspectives of the training methods usually used, have a great impact on the decision-making of CDSS in the clinic, which is also the reason why clinicians do not agree much with the decision results of CDSS. An algorithm that can accurately detect medical images of skin cancer also has physicians who support the accuracy of the diagnosis. However, black box algorithms are opaque, which means that physicians cannot account for how the algorithm got its recommendation or arrived at its diagnosis. This poses a challenge for clinical work: do we have enough reason to trust a diagnostically opaque algorithm when we cannot establish how it obtained the diagnosis? How should physicians handle difficult-to-understand diagnoses? Can doctors be responsible for medical diagnoses with AI systems that they cannot understand?

3.2 Diagnostic Accuracy Issues

In real medical diagnosis, physicians are often confronted with a myriad of complex information, but in many trials, the conditions under which AI performs diagnosis are isolated, and overall, there is very little AI that actually penetrates deep into the clinical process. Studies that include as much additional information as a real clinical setting diagnosis are minimal. The presentation of trial results is also not fully objective, and most studies do not list missing data, a situation that would affect the accuracy of trial results. Due to the insufficient number of reliable studies, the fact that there are still too few relevant data and the inadequacy of the trial design, it is too early to make assertions about the medical diagnostic capabilities of AI to draw final conclusions in a real-world setting. Knowing the impact of AI on patient recovery outcomes requires the design of randomized clinical trials with alternative medical protocols, and no such trials have yet been able to examine the performance of AI in terms of timely treatment, patient discharge time, and survival rates. Few studies have been able to provide externally validated results or compare the performance of deep learning models and physicians using the same sample. In addition, the prevalence of poor reporting in deep learning studies limits the reliable interpretation of reported diagnostic accuracy.

In purely technical aspects (e.g., algorithm performance and accuracy) AI still performs remarkably well, but in close clinical application scenarios, it is challenging to turn physician experience and knowledge into replicable digital procedures. For example, pathology diagnosis mode is presented in the form of images, most easily based on big data for diagnosis and differential diagnosis of diseases through pattern recognition. Currently, in pathology, AI has been applied to assist in the diagnosis of hematologic malignancies (mainly leukemia). However, there are still limitations to the application of AI in pathology, as pathological solid tumor parenchyma and mesenchymal components are more complex, and the confirmation of the diagnosis of some tumors also relies on immunohistochemistry, all of which will greatly increase the difficulty of AI diagnosis.

Moreover, most intelligent diagnostic products do not fully follow the clinical workflow links. Taking lung nodule diagnosis as an example, it is not a problem to just diagnose a lung nodule, but not to determine whether there are other diseases, and the consequences of misdiagnosis or omission are very serious. The current medical aid system is only responsible for finding out the lesion, and the final characterization is done by the physician. Take imaging artificial intelligence, which is currently most widely used in clinical practice, as an example. To determine whether a patient has pneumonia through X-ray films, an imaging physician cannot make a diagnosis based on the films alone. The most an imaging doctor can say after reading the film is "this lung X-ray is consistent with pneumonia signs given the typical clinical symptoms." It is likely that different imaging specialists will have different opinions about what the images show. The reason is that an image consistent with pneumonia may also appear to be an incomplete lung expansion. Pneumonia may seem simple, but the final diagnosis requires a combination of the patient's clinical history, symptoms, blood tests, and images. Another more realistic case is illustrative. A well-known hospital in Shenzhen diagnosed a child with nodular lung manifestations through the Intelligent Companion System. If diagnosed and treated according to the CDSS, there is a possibility of overdiagnosis and over treatment. Meanwhile, the diagnostic criteria and treatment responsibility become a problem for continued research.

3.3 Problems with Diagnostic Criteria

The rigor and iterative nature of medical knowledge and the complexity of the disease that cannot be predicted precisely make the design of CDSS need to consider more factors. In addition to the multiple factors of the patients themselves, countless new data have to be screened, updated, and supplemented in real time. In the medical field alone, a large number of clinical findings need to be constantly understood by scientists and engineers developing CDSS, and old content has to be removed, and the core is to select high-quality evidence for CDSS, which is also a problem for CDSS developers. In the current research environment, few research teams have evaluated the efficacy of CDSS and thought about it, which means that the practicality of the system has not been evaluated by the industry, and it can even be said that there is no accurate data on clinical efficacy, and we cannot get the authoritative evaluation index and standard, which will largely affect the standardized use of CDSS in the clinical setting.

The existing problems of CDSS and the complexity of the clinical workflow make the integration of the two more difficult. It is also important to consider that some CDSS that need to be used online cannot be used in the hospital due to the logical or physical isolation of the network in different levels and conditions of the hospital.

3.4 Responsibility of CDSS

CDSS takes implementation action plans based on established algorithms. Artificial intelligence has been given more autonomy and has been added to human social behavior with a unique individual "consciousness" and has been given more power in the medical decision-making process, but also inevitably more responsibility.

The Medical Device Classification Catalogue issued by the State Drug Administration in 2022 indicates that medical AI products that only give clinical diagnostic advice through the support of algorithms and have only an auxiliary diagnostic role rather than directly making a conclusive diagnosis need to be managed in accordance with the regulations for Class II medical devices. If it is a medical AI product that automatically identifies lesion sites through algorithms and provides clear diagnostic conclusion hints on this basis, it needs to be regulated according to the management regulations of Class III medical devices because of its escalated application risks.

We cannot avoid the attribution of responsibility, and in the conventional medical world the dominant position of doctors is unshakeable. But when CDSS is applied widely in the clinical practice, its performance and reliability highlight its role in routine and critical clinical events, which may somehow diminish the doctors' status in the medical service, and at the same time, the doctor's medical behavior will also be trivialized. Subesequently, for patients, especially those who may have suffered medical violations, the perspective of recourse against the medical party should be more biased toward the CDSS. Such an understanding has caused a lot of controversies, whether it is philosophical, ethical theoretical analysis, or jurisprudential application of thinking, the vast majority of scholars when discussing the issue of attribution of responsibility focus on the medical treatment or should the doctor be responsible for the argument. If CDSS is involved in the scope of the responsible subject, we cannot avoid the problems of responsibility arising, and the responsible parties passing the buck to each other, and the division of power and responsibility being confused, which threatens patients' health, rights, consistency of social moral framework, and clarity of legal responsibility. The Management Specification for Artificial Intelligence-Assisted Diagnostic Technology (2017 Edition) clarifies the positioning of medical AI-assisted diagnostic technology: an auxiliary diagnostic and clinical decision support system. The conclusion of medical AI-aided diagnosis technology cannot be directly used as the conclusion of the final clinical diagnosis, but only as one of the reference bases for clinical diagnosis. Only the conclusion of qualified clinicians can be used as the final diagnosis. However, the development of decision-making will change with the continuous improvement of technology, and the objective and rational evaluation criteria need to be improved gradually.

3.5 The Problem of Shared Decision-Making and Patient Autonomy

The prerequisite for the exercise of patient autonomy is shared decision-making. In clinical treatment and medical ethical practice, patients have the right to adopt medical measures and accept medical actions according to their own wishes, and they also have the right to decide whether to accept medical advice or not. On this basis, in order for the patient's consent to be valid in medical services, the doctor needs to inform the patient in advance, truthfully, and adequately; and the patient can participate in clinical shared decision-making only after fully understanding the actual content and impact of medical processes and medical actions. Thus, it can be seen that comprehensible disclosure of medical information and medical practices is very important.

Take the Watson Oncology Diagnostic System as an example: this system uses "maximizing survival time" as a clinical goal and provides recommendations for treatment options (McDougall 2018). This gives rise to the problem that the treatment plan may not be determined by the individual patient's wishes but by the conclusions driven by the philosophy of the CDSS algorithm. This will lead to the inequality of medical information between doctors and patients or even the loss of medical decision-making power of patients, or even the dominance of a paternalistic decision-making model driven by medical artificial intelligence, which is a regression of the diagnosis and treatment model and philosophy.

When considering the weight of medical treatment decisions, the Watson Oncology Diagnostic System takes the maximization of the patient's survival time as the primary and most important consideration criterion. If the patient expects the least pain, it will be difficult for the algorithm to help achieve it. This can also illustrate that if medical AI is included in the control of medical decision-making, various rights/dignity of patients will be subverted and destroyed. Considering the long-term development perspective, medical AI that fails to address the issue of patient's free will realization in its development will inevitably bring about individual harm. At present, it is difficult for CDSS to weigh the most appropriate medical behavior and the best medical outcome from the patient's perspective, and the algorithm of CDSS rarely involves the multi-dimensional rights of patients during treatment, while the real specific medical process should be the maximum integration (including technical, ethical, and legal issues), and the treatment decision made entirely by machine autonomy is a violation of human freedom rights, breaking the key principle of traditional medicine "patient-centered." The "patient-centered" principle of traditional medicine is broken. The Code of Practice for the Management of Artificial Intelligence-Assisted Diagnostic Techniques

(2017 Edition) also clearly explains how it should be used in clinical practice and its precautions.

4 Specialized Application of CDSS

4.1 CDSS in the Diagnosis of Rare Diseases

Rare diseases are a group of diseases with very low incidence, also known as orphan diseases. The World Health Organization defines rare diseases as diseases that affect 0.65–1 per 1000 of the total population, with a total of about 8000 diseases affecting about 400 million people worldwide. Rare diseases are mostly genetic diseases, some of which are caused by severe mutations in a single gene, which also makes them generally more severe. Because rare diseases are numerous and diverse, most healthcare workers have little exposure to them, and a lack of knowledge about specific rare diseases can lead to missed diagnoses, making the search for care a long and tortuous experience for most patients.

The CDSS is expected to bring the experience of rare disease diagnosis and treatment to the frontline clinical workflow, and provide diagnostic advice for rare diseases to physicians without interrupting their work at hand.

Existing rare disease CDSS can generally be classified as knowledge base based, machine learning based, and online retrieval based. The main difference between the three is that they rely on the existing knowledge base system or rely on machine learning models for prediction.

Knowledge base-based CDSS provides clinical decision aids with the help of existing knowledge base and uses retrieval and big data technologies. The main difference between existing knowledge base-based CDSS is the knowledge base used and the difference in analysis engines. The knowledge bases can be broadly classified into existing public knowledge bases, Electronic Medical Record (EMR) mining knowledge, literature mining knowledge, etc.; the algorithmic principles of their analytic engines can be broadly classified into machine learning-based methods or information retrieval-type methods.

Phenomizer (Köhler et al. 2009) measures the phenotypic similarity between patients to be seen and genetic cases annotated in HPO by adjusting semantic similarity metrics, giving similarity scores for similar diseases and calculating p-values with statistical models. This method outperforms term-matching methods that do not consider semantic relationships between terms, especially for cases that contain phenotypic noise or inaccurate clinical descriptions. In contrast, DECIPHER (Bragin et al. 2013) is an interactive web-based database that contains a set of tools designed to help interpret genomic variation and contains more than 30,000 rare disease cases contributed by 270 centers for clinicians to share and compare phenotypic and genotypic data.

In addition to phenotypic data, a full comparison of patient characteristics requires the inclusion of more important information such as exomes and genomes, which has led to the emergence of a series of CDSS that combine phenotypic and genotypic decision-making, such as GeneYenta, GeneMatcher, GenIO, and PhenomeCentral. These tools are accessible online and use HPO terms for matching, and the latter two can upload gene files in VCF format. Most tools, when analyzed, can output a rare disease match score to aid in clinical decision-making.

With the accumulation of EMRs, a large number of machine learning CDSS based on clinical case mining have emerged. However, since such systems are more difficult to interpret the derivation process, most clinicians utilize them for research model exploration rather than direct use in clinical practice for reliability and accountability reasons. Therefore, most of the current machine learning-based rare disease CDSS are in the prototype stage, mostly not deployed on the Internet, and most of them make predictions for a specific few rare diseases, which are more difficult to apply to clinical prediction scenarios for all rare diseases.

According to whether rare disease CDSSs output diagnostic results, they can be classified into explicit and implicit. Unlike the above two types of CDSS, some search tools do not directly output prediction results but assist physicians to search online to find relevant case information, which also belongs to the broad CDSS. Clinically, for complex patient cases, clinicians usually look for peer-researched patient cases with similar characteristics in the literature such as case reports. However, conventional search engines usually optimize queries for certain high-frequency keywords and make recommendations based on popularity (e.g., recommending literature that is more frequently visited), a search method that favors more user viewing is less meaningful for rare disease searches. As a result, the process is often time-consuming and inefficient, and physicians need an online search tool to assist in finding patients with similar clinical characteristics.

The rare disease search tool FindZebra (Svenstrup et al. 2015) is similar to other search engines, but its data sources mainly use OMIM, GARD, Orphanet, Wikipedia, etc. FindZebra was compared with other online search tools google.com, pubmed.gov, omim.org, etc., and web searches of 56 diagnosed rare disease cases were conducted using each of these tools. It was found that the recall rate of rare diseases was significantly higher in FindZebra. In contrast, the work of Taboada et al. (2014) focused on semantic indexing of case reports in the literature, which can be retrieved from PubMed's patient case summaries. Both of these can provide matching results from the literature base based on the input symptoms. In addition, Porat et al. (2014) noticed that existing DPAs do not contain any prenatal patient characteristics, and DPAs based on postnatal patients cannot be applied in prenatal diagnosis. For this reason, they proposed a web-based, searchable genetic disease database for prenatal diagnosis. Unlike the CDS for postnatal rare diseases, it does not rely on traditional DPAs, but rather summarizes 329 sets of proven "prenatal ultrasound phenotype-syndrome associations" from the extensive literature. Their study also provides a new perspective on the diagnosis of rare diseases.

4.2 CDSS in Diabetes Management

There is a lifelong and complex nature of diabetes management, and its burden has severely impacted national health and even economic development. On the one hand, diabetes requires long-term, even lifelong medication, which implies significant direct medical expenditures, while the rejuvenation of its complications severely affects the ability of the workforce to contribute to society. On the other hand, the existing diabetes management model requires close collaboration between community general practitioners, diabetes specialists, and related health professionals, adding significant human resources and management costs on top of the cost of medicine. Long-term effective diabetes management is particularly difficult in regions with relatively backward socioeconomic and medical resource development. How to effectively improve the efficiency of medical services has become a pressing issue in China's medical field today.

The development of information technology, artificial intelligence, big data, and evidence-based medicine in recent years has brought hope for the improvement of the efficiency of medical services. Among them, CDSS based on electronic health record (EHR) is one of the important solutions to solve this core problem (Osheroff 2012; Greenes 2014). There are many technical routes to realize CDSS, among which CDSS based on an ontology knowledge base is undoubtedly one of the most rigorous and scalable solutions recognized around the world (McGuinness 2023; Conway et al. 2017). In recent years, CDSS products have emerged, including many projects for primary and inpatient diabetes, but CDSS for diabetes using ontologies as a knowledge base source are relatively limited and their concept is still relatively unknown today.

CDSS has a large heterogeneity in their frameworks and can be classified into quizzer, EHR, sensor, and multimodal fusion based on the information collection input side.

Q&A-based CDSS uses user-initiated entry of information as the information input side. Its inputters can be patients, doctors, other healthcare providers, and multiple users, and the application scenario can be hospital consultation or patient self-management at home. The information collected is combined with the developed question-answer ontology to form standardized and structured patient information, which is then converted to the format required by the reasoner in the Java engine and fed into the reasoner, which combines the data, knowledge base and inference rules and reasons to generate conclusions. The efficiency and accuracy of patient information collection are highly dependent on the question setting and the quality of the user's answers. The entry of structured information simplifies the processing of input information but may make it more difficult for users to use. In particular, there is a lot of decision-making information affecting diabetic patients, including blood glucose monitoring and lifestyle information in addition to basic demographic information, all of which make it more difficult for clinicians and patients to enter information. Unstructured information, such as natural language and scanned copies of checklists, requires data standardization and structuring through certain techniques corresponding to the response ontology. This input simplifies and facilitates user use, but increases the difficulty of information recognition. Therefore, the setting of questions and quizzers by a research team consisting of clinical, medical information, computer science, and clinical epidemiology experts is essential to improve the use and user experience of CDSS. Among the published ontology-based CDSS, Chen et al. (2012) captured less variety of patient information through physician input of patient information. Onto Diabetic (2016) (Sherimon and Krishnan 2015) and IRS-T2D (2016) (Mahmoud and Elbeh 2016), on the other hand, require more data information to be entered by the user. Chen et al. (2017) introduce a temporal dimension of information on top of this, which greatly enriches the input information, but also poses some challenges to the ease of use for the user. Information entry in these CDSS often occurs during the doctor–patient communication process, which makes it easier for physicians to synthesize the actual situation, values, and preferences of patients. Some CDSS (Chen et al. 2017) use a fuzzy algorithm to calculate personalized glycated hemoglobin control targets and a TOPSIS algorithm to consider multidimensional factors to comprehensively evaluate medication regimens and give a ranking of recommended drugs. However, these CDSS inputs are highly dependent on adequate physician and patient communication and accuracy of information entry. Diabetic patients have a large amount of medical information including blood glucose monitoring records, and it is difficult to comprehensively capture patient information based only on user entry methods.

In medical institutions with well-established EHR or electronic medical record (EMR) systems, a large amount of information about diabetes visits is recorded in detail and stored in a standardized manner. The EHR-based CDSS is designed to directly import the patient's health data in the hospital, including demographic information, vital signs, comorbidities and complications, laboratory tests, medication prescriptions, radiology reports, and surgical records, by interfacing the EHR with the CDSS input. el-SAPPAGH et al. have designed DDO (before 2015) (El-Sappagh and Ali 2016), DMTO (2015) (El-Sappagh et al. 2018), and FASTO (2018) (El-Sappagh et al. 2019). DDO is used for the diagnosis of diabetes, DMTO is the most complete ontology for the treatment of type 2 diabetes, and FASTO is used for the real-time management of insulin in diabetic patients, especially in type 1 diabetes. Among them, FASTO is an extension of DMTO and DDO. Its biggest update is the inclusion of rules for insulin dose adjustment, and other domain knowledge and rules have been optimized and expanded to varying degrees. In addition, FASTO specifies a standard model for patient data interface as FHIR standard (providing protocols and standards for communication between different systems), which can support the development of mobile health applications, clinical decision support systems on cloud environments, and interoperability between distributed EHRs, mobile devices, and wireless regional networks. However, it is currently only for type 1 diabetes and its clinical application is greatly limited. In addition, it lacks treatment protocols for different clinical scenarios, diet protocols with multiple essential dietary nutrients, and user-friendly units of measurement, as does DMTO. OMDP (2019) (Chen et al. 2019) adds knowledge of genes and diabetes typing to integrate prevention, screening, and treatment compared to FASTO and DMTO. However, it does not currently publish details of the model for standardizing the patient data interface and the conversion from raw EHR data to data available to the inference engine.

The sensor-based CDSS collects patient data by interfacing with sensors through the inputs. The sensors can provide real-time patient monitoring data, including vital signs, blood glucose, and blood glucose fluctuation trajectories under real-time monitoring based on wearable devices. The literature shows that blood glucose fluctuations have a significant impact on both the onset and prognosis of diabetes, so the data from the connected sensors will help the CDSS to derive an effective treatment plan. Currently, semantic sensor network ontology (SSN) is a W3C-recommended ontology for describing sensor observations, processes, features, samples, observed properties, and actuators. Health level 7 FHIR standard can also provide standards for transforming patient sensor data, EHR data, and knowledge ontologies to understand each other and operate together. FASTO describes methods and details of sensor-based CDSS construction.

4.3 CDSS in Anesthesia Management

An important application of information technology in medical quality management is CDSS. Through CDSS tools, intelligent reminders of certain key aspects of work are realized in an embedded way, including behavior monitoring, execution reminding, and result tracking, which eventually form a closed-loop management of the medical process and realize continuous improvement of medical quality. Through the whole process, active and closed-loop quality management, and the medical anesthesia process that has been analyzed, summarized, and optimized will be solidified by information technology to realize medical behavior.

Anesthesia records are the main component of clinical anesthesia work, and patient perioperative data can provide references for subsequent anesthesia treatment and case management. The current AIMS in major hospitals can collect data from sources such as monitors, hospital information systems, ventilators, and anesthesia workstations in real time. The anesthesiologist records the patient's fluid balance status, surgery, medication records, special events, and other information in real time according to intraoperative anesthesia management, so the anesthesia record is a comprehensive database of real-time information during the patient's surgery.

With the increasing popularity of AIMS (anesthesia information management system), researchers have used machine learning to comprehensively analyze the comprehensive database of patient anesthesia and develop a hardware system, CDSS, that provides real-time decision aids for anesthesiologists to reduce physician errors. The system mainly collects data from AIMS, categorizes the data into usable data by transformation, filtering, and missing fill, and the decision processor applies algorithms to the data and determines whether to notify or alert (e.g., pop-up messages or flashing buttons) on the AIMS according to the decision rules that have been set. In the early days, CDSS was mainly used for routine workflow reminders, such as prompting physicians to give intraoperative antibiotics, beta-blockers, optimize ventilator parameters, avoid wasting anesthetic drugs, and check anesthesia bills. The CDSS can also be used to identify pediatric traumatic brain injury patients undergoing neurosurgery, identify the target population based on patient information from AIMS, and remind anesthesiologists of the key anesthetic points to focus on intraoperatively according to the set algorithm rules, reducing the incidence of intraoperative adverse events. However, the reminder interface of the early CDSS is monotonous and sometimes difficult to attract anesthesiologists' attention. The new CDSS integrates the patient's circulatory indexes, respiratory parameters, fluid balance, laboratory test results, and alarm reminders in a single reminder interface with different colored organ dynamic diagrams, which comprehensively and vividly reflects the patient's intraoperative situation and improves the efficiency of anesthesiologists' perioperative management.

Most of the current CDSS are reactive support systems. Researchers developing new systems can collect data from monitors directly while processing large amounts of data streams with the help of 5G networks to develop CDSS with real-time prediction, but such predictive CDSS are still in the research stage.

Information systems can also achieve a higher level of intelligence by embedding clinical knowledge into the processes we work with through CDSS tools. Specific features include:

1. Automated prompts for operation specifications: When a certain anesthesia modality is selected, the system can automatically pop up a standardized operation guide with illustrations and reminders of key considerations. This reminder can be linked to the qualification of anesthesiologists, for very senior and skilled anesthesiologists, the system cannot prompt, but for anesthesiologists with insufficient practice, the system will automatically pop up a reminder, effectively guiding the standardized clinical operation (Nair et al. 2017).
2. Automatic warning of hypothermia: The output of the monitor for the data of key vital signs can reach a frequency of 15 s/group of data. If based on clinical experience, hypothermia can be classified into different danger levels, such as 36 °C, 35.5 °C, and 35 °C, and also the duration after reaching the numerical standard can be defined. In this way, it can be automatically collected by a computer and assisted by the clinic for early warning, and necessary measures can be taken as soon as possible to reduce the possibility of dangerous events.
3. Data integration and sharing: The information of surgical anesthesia is integrated with the preoperative and postoperative clinical information, and the cases that require longer observation of various complications, such as intravertebral anesthesia, general anesthesia tracheal intubation, and central venous puncture, can be automatically reminded and entered in the postoperative department, thus ensuring the integrity and continuity of the data.

5 Summary

CDSS can greatly improve the efficiency of clinicians and help them to grasp individualized information about patients more quickly. The performance of CDSS currently in use varies, and it is beneficial to discuss and summarize the problems of existing CDSS to promote further development and improvement of the system.

5.1 Clinical Problems of CDSS

1. The CDSS was developed to assist physicians in clinical diagnosis and treatment, but the following problems exist in the experience of healthcare professionals: some physicians think that the use of CDSS hinders the communication between physicians and patients, and worry that the system affects the ability of physicians to think independently in the clinical process and make decisions in unexpected situations.
2. The concept and purpose of CDSS are of high R&D value, but the reasons for the unsatisfactory promotion and use in practice include: (1) difficulty of use, ignoring the simplicity of human–computer interaction during use by physicians; (2) insufficient humanization of system design; (3) low compatibility of CDSS with current medical systems.

3. Insufficient utilization of historical data by existing CDSS: (1) the data volume of a single medical institution cannot meet the coverage of the CDSS model, but the establishment of a cloud database on a large scale involves the confidentiality and privacy of medical data, and the case data format of different medical institutions is not uniform and the structure is complicated, which reduces the computational capacity of the system; (2) most of the patient data processing is horizontal comparison, and the coverage of the longitudinal nature of the data is incomplete, which leads to different opinions when the system reformulates the treatment plan for new clinical information; (3) the existence of misdiagnosis or nonoptimal prescription cases may be applied to the next medical diagnosis.

5.2 Prospects for the Future Development of CDSS

In order to improve the design of CDSS and promote the application of new systems to better assist clinicians in diagnosis and treatment, we propose the future development outlook from three key aspects of clinical use, system technology, and medical data, taking into account the current typical application systems.

1. From the perspective of clinician use: (1) clinicians participate in the design and development of CDSS during the R&D stage to improve the practicality of the system and reduce physicians' distrust of the system's decision-making; (2) the system is designed to be more user friendly, providing clinicians with decision-making solutions along with corresponding medical explanations; and (3) training for clinicians on the use of the system with corresponding operation manuals and other training materials.
2. From the perspective of system technology: (1) realize the "dual-engine" knowledge source, i.e., the combination of evidence-based medical knowledge base + hospital clinical database can better face various clinical diseases; (2) research classification or regression algorithms with low computational cost and fast computational speed can realize efficient solution giving while ensuring the accuracy of decision-making; (3) for when there are many clinical features in the patient data set, the data can be grouped by using principal component analysis (PCA) to reduce the dimensionality or diagnosis related groups (DRG) to speed up the efficiency of data mining.
3. In the use of medical data: (1) CDSS should achieve real-time interaction with physicians to obtain dynamic patient characteristics and attributes, and develop more personalized treatment plans through longitudinal comparison; (2) CDSS implementation needs to be integrated with hospital information system (HIS) to share clinical data, accelerate the treatment process, and improve the efficiency of hospital work and services; (3) the amount of historical data must be large enough and include various rare diseases and special cases so that the system can improve the accuracy and success rate based on the modeling. By optimizing the CDSS, it can make its decision-making scheme more practical in the actual hospital environment, provide clinicians with theoretical and data-backed recommendations, and assist clinicians in improving their ability to achieve high-quality and safe clinical treatment.

References

Afzal M, Hussain M, Ali T, Hussain J, Khan W, Lee S, et al. Knowledge-based query construction using the CDSS knowledge base for efficient evidence retrieval. Sensors. 2015;15(9):21294–314.

Allard M. Overcoming cultural barriers to the adoption of object technology. Inf Syst Manag. 1998;15(3):82–5.

Ambinder EP. A history of the shift toward full computerization of medicine. J Oncol Pract. 2005;1(2):54–6.

Arooj S, Sur R, Imran A, Almuhaimeed A, Alzahrani AK, Alzahrani A. A deep convolutional neural network for the early detection of heart disease. Biomedicine. 2022;10(11):2796.

Ayaz A, Yanartaş M. An analysis on the unified theory of acceptance and use of technology theory (UTAUT): acceptance of electronic document man-

agement system (EDMS). Comput Hum Behav Rep. 2020;2:100032.
Bandyopadhyay K, Barnes C. An analysis of factors affecting user acceptance of ERP systems in the United States. Int J Human Capital Information Technol Professionals. 2012;3(1):1–14.
Belard A, Buchman T, Forsberg J, Potter BK, Dente CJ, Kirk A, et al. Precision diagnosis: a view of the clinical decision support systems (CDSS) landscape through the lens of critical care. J Clin Monit Comput. 2016;31(2):261–71.
Bragin E, Chatzimichali EA, Wright CF, Hurles ME, Firth HV, Bevan AP, et al. Decipher: database for the interpretation of phenotype-linked plausibly pathogenic sequence and copy-number variation. Nucleic Acids Res. 2013;42(D1):D993–D1000.
Braun V, Clarke V. Using thematic analysis in psychology. Qual Res Psychol. 2006;3(2):77–101.
Cabana MD, Rand CS, Powe NR, Wu AW, Wilson MH, Abboud P-AC, et al. Why don't physicians follow clinical practice guidelines? JAMA. 1999;282(15):1458.
Camacho J, Zanoletti-Mannello M, Landis-Lewis Z, Kane-Gill SL, Boyce RD. A conceptual framework to study the implementation of clinical decision support systems (BEAR): literature review and concept mapping. J Med Internet Res. 2020;22(8):e18388.
Catho G, Centemero NS, Catho H, Ranzani A, Balmelli C, Landelle C, et al. Factors determining the adherence to antimicrobial guidelines and the adoption of computerised decision support systems by physicians: a qualitative study in three European hospitals. Int J Med Inform. 2020;141:104233.
Chen R-C, Huang Y-H, Bau C-T, Chen S-M. A recommendation system based on domain ontology and SWRL for anti-diabetic drugs selection. Expert Syst Appl. 2012;39(4):3995–4006.
Chen R-C, Jiang HQ, Huang C-Y, Bau C-T. Clinical decision support system for diabetes based on ontology reasoning and TOPSIS analysis. J Healthc Eng. 2017;2017:1–14.
Chen L, Lu D, Zhu M, Muzammal M, Samuel OW, Huang G, et al. OMDP: an ontology-based model for diagnosis and treatment of diabetes patients in remote healthcare systems. Int J Distributed Sensor Networks. 2019;15(5):155014771984711.
Cho YI, Johnson TP, VanGeest JB. Enhancing surveys of health care professionals. Eval Health Prof. 2013;36(3):382–407.
Chow AL, Ang A, Chow CZ, Ng TM, Teng C, Ling LM, et al. Implementation hurdles of an interactive, integrated, point-of-care computerised decision support system for hospital antibiotic prescription. Int J Antimicrob Agents. 2016;47(2):132–9.
Chung P, Scandlyn J, Dayan PS, Mistry RD. Working at the intersection of context, culture, and technology: provider perspectives on antimicrobial stewardship in the emergency department using electronic health record clinical decision support. Am J Infect Control. 2017;45(11):1198–202.
Conway N, Adamson KA, Cunningham SG, Emslie Smith A, Nyberg P, Smith BH, et al. Decision support for diabetes in Scotland: implementation and evaluation of a clinical decision support system. J Diabetes Sci Technol. 2017;12(2):381–8.
Corbin JM, Strauss AL. Basics of qualitative research: techniques and procedures for developing grounded theory. Los Angeles: SAGE; 2015.
DeLone WH, McLean ER. Measuring e-commerce success: applying the delone & amp; McLean information systems success model. Int J Electron Commer. 2004;9(1):31–47.
El-Sappagh S, Ali F. DDO: a diabetes mellitus diagnosis ontology. Appl Inform. 2016;3(1):5.
El-Sappagh S, Kwak D, Ali F, Kwak K-S. DMTO: a realistic ontology for standard diabetes mellitus treatment. J Biomed Semantics. 2018;9(1):8.
El-Sappagh S, Ali F, Hendawi A, Jang J-H, Kwak K-S. A mobile health monitoring-and-treatment system based on integration of the SSN sensor ontology and the HL7 FHIR standard. BMC Med Inform Decis Mak. 2019;19(1):97.
Goud R, van Engen-Verheul M, de Keizer NF, Bal R, Hasman A, Hellemans IM, et al. The effect of computerized decision support on barriers to guideline implementation: a qualitative study in outpatient cardiac rehabilitation. Int J Med Inform. 2010;79(6):430–7.
Greenes RA. Clinical decision support: the road to broad adoption. Amsterdam: Academic Press/Elsevier; 2014.
Huang C, Huang X, Fang Y, Xu J, Qu Y, Zhai P, et al. Sample imbalance disease classification model based on association rule feature selection. Pattern Recogn Lett. 2020;133:280–6.
Jung SY, Hwang H, Lee K, Lee H-Y, Kim E, Kim M, et al. Barriers and facilitators to implementation of medication decision support systems in electronic medical records: mixed methods approach based on structural equation modeling and qualitative analysis. JMIR Med Inform. 2020;8(7):e18758.
Khairat S, Marc D, Crosby W, Al SA. Reasons for physicians not adopting clinical decision support systems: critical analysis (preprint). JMIR Med Inform. 2018;6:e24.
Kilsdonk E, Peute LW, Jaspers MWM. Factors influencing implementation success of guideline-based clinical decision support systems: a systematic review and gaps analysis. Int J Med Inform. 2017;98:56–64.
Köhler S, Schulz MH, Krawitz P, Bauer S, Dölken S, Ott CE, et al. Clinical diagnostics in human genetics with semantic similarity searches in ontologies. Am J Hum Genet. 2009;85(4):457–64.
Kortteisto T, Komulainen J, Mäkelä M, Kunnamo I, Kaila M. Clinical decision support must be useful, functional is not enough: a qualitative study of computer-based clinical decision support in primary care. BMC Health Serv Res. 2012;12(1):349.
Lai F, Macmillan J, Daudelin DH, Kent DM. The potential of training to increase acceptance and use of computerized decision support systems for medical diagnosis. Hum Factors. 2006;48(1):95–108.

Laka M, Milazzo A, Merlin T. Factors that impact the adoption of clinical decision support systems (CDSS) for antibiotic management. Int J Environ Res Public Health. 2021;18(4):1901.

Leslie SJ, Hartswood M, Meurig C, McKee SP, Slack R, Procter R, et al. Clinical decision support software for management of chronic heart failure: development and evaluation. Comput Biol Med. 2006;36(5):495–506.

Liberati EG, Ruggiero F, Galuppo L, Gorli M, González-Lorenzo M, Maraldi M, et al. What hinders the uptake of computerized decision support systems in hospitals? A qualitative study and framework for implementation. Implement Sci. 2017;12(1):113.

Lugtenberg M, Pasveer D, van der Weijden T, Westert GP, Kool RB. Exposure to and experiences with a computerized decision support intervention in primary care: results from a process evaluation. BMC Fam Pract. 2015a;16(1):141.

Lugtenberg M, Weenink J-W, van der Weijden T, Westert GP, Kool RB. Implementation of multiple-domain covering computerized decision support systems in primary care: a focus group study on perceived barriers. BMC Med Inform Decis Mak. 2015b;15(1):82.

Mahmoud N, Elbeh H. IRS-T2D. Proceedings of the 10th international conference on informatics and systems; 2016. p. 203–9.

McDougall RJ. Computer knows best? The need for value-flexibility in medical AI. J Med Ethics. 2018;45(3):156–60.

Deborah L. McGuinness. Ontology development 101: a guide to creating your first ontology [Internet]. 2023. http://ksl.stanford.edu/people/dlm/papers/ontology-tutorial-noy-mcguinness-abstract.html.

Moxey A, Robertson J, Newby D, Hains I, Williamson M, Pearson S-A. Computerized clinical decision support for prescribing: provision does not guarantee uptake. J Am Med Inform Assoc. 2010;17(1):25–33.

Nair BG, Gabel E, Hofer I, Schwid HA, Cannesson M. Intraoperative clinical decision support for anesthesia. Anesth Analg. 2017;124(2):603–17.

Osheroff JA. Improving outcomes with clinical decision support: an implementer's guide. Chicago: HIMSS; 2012.

Ozkaynak M, Wu D, Hannah K, Dayan P, Mistry R. Examining workflow in a pediatric emergency department to develop a clinical decision support for an antimicrobial stewardship program. Appl Clin Inform. 2018;09(02):248–60.

Porat S, de Rham M, Giamboni D, Van Mieghem T, Baud D. Phenotip – a web-based instrument to help diagnosing fetal syndromes antenatally. Orphanet J Rare Dis. 2014;9(1):204.

Sherimon PC, Krishnan R. Ontodiabetic: an ontology-based clinical decision support system for diabetic patients. Arab J Sci Eng. 2015;41(3):1145–60.

Shibl R, Lawley M, Debuse J. Factors influencing decision support system acceptance. Decis Support Syst. 2013;54(2):953–61.

Short D, Frischer M, Bashford J. The development and evaluation of a computerised decision support system for primary care based upon 'patient profile decision analysis'. J Innov Health Inform. 2003;11(4):195–202.

Sutton RT, Pincock D, Baumgart DC, Sadowski DC, Fedorak RN, Kroeker KI. An overview of clinical decision support systems: benefits, risks, and strategies for success. NPJ Digit Med. 2020;3(1):17.

Svenstrup D, Jørgensen HL, Winther O. Rare disease diagnosis: a review of web search, social media and large-scale data-mining approaches. Rare Dis. 2015;3(1):e1083145.

Taboada M, Rodríguez H, Martínez D, Pardo M, Sobrido MJ. Automated semantic annotation of rare disease cases: a case study. Database. 2014;2014:1–13.

Trivedi MH, Kern JK, Marcee A, Grannemann B, Kleiber B, Bettinger T, et al. Development and implementation of computerized clinical guidelines: barriers and solutions. Methods Inf Med. 2002;41(05):435–42.

Tsiknakis M, Kouroubali A. Organizational factors affecting successful adoption of innovative eHealth services: a case study employing the FITT framework. Int J Med Inform. 2009;78(1):39–52.

Yao W, Kumar A. CONFlexFlow: integrating flexible clinical pathways into clinical decision support systems using context and rules. Decis Support Syst. 2013;55(2):499–515.

Yusof MM, Kuljis J, Papazafeiropoulou A, Stergioulas LK. An evaluation framework for health information systems: human, organization and technology-fit factors (hot-fit). Int J Med Inform. 2008;77(6):386–98.

Zuiderwijk A, Janssen M, Dwivedi YK. Acceptance and use predictors of open data technologies: drawing upon the unified theory of acceptance and use of technology. Gov Inf Q. 2015;32(4):429–40.

Artificial Intelligence in Clinical Skills Training and Assessment in Anesthesiology

Hong Jiang

Researches on the application of artificial intelligence (AI) in clinical training and assessment have only emerged in recent years, as a result of the development and advancement of AI technology. Though it has been a global trend, different countries took different features in their exploration of this topic. In China, researchers are more concerned about the integration of AI with the utilization of clinical technologies to reduce the workload of healthcare professionals and improve the efficiency of skill training, while related research in other countries focuses on the revelation of the current state of how AI participating and assisting medical education, including the promotion of instruction's assessment, and how both instructors and students review AI's participation in their teaching and learning process.

1 The Application of AI in Anesthesiology Clinical Skills Training and Assessment in China

AI is changing various aspects of clinical skill training and assessment in anesthesiology. On one hand, technologies such as "real-time collection and identification of multi-source clinical teaching data," "analysis of teaching indicators for AI methods and construction of prediction and warning model," "teaching evaluation algorithm and intelligent teaching intervention hint" can track and analyze students' performance and provide advice for improvement automatically (Bin et al. 2019). On the other hand, against the backdrop of the COVID-19 pandemic, activities of all kinds are somehow halted and may be suspended at any time. Using AI to score students' performance on both written and in-person components of clinical skills assessment is promising and efficient. Researchers show their confidence in the positive future of the application of AI expert systems in students' training, anesthesia teaching, and hospital development.

H. Jiang (✉)
Department of Anesthesiology, Shanghai Ninth People's Hospital, Shanghai Jiao Tong University School of Medicine, Shanghai, China

1.1 Overview of the Application of AI in Medical Education

With the continuous advancement of technologies, the application of AI in medical education has become feasible, and the application models often used are collecting data (anesthesia operation procedures), constructing data sets (standard operations), modeling with AI statistical analysis tools (evaluation), and establishing training evaluation and analysis systems (control validation).

The actual applications are as follows:

M. Xia, H. Jiang (eds.), *Artificial Intelligence in Anesthesiology*,
https://doi.org/10.1007/978-981-99-5925-9_11

1. Intelligent Assessment and Evaluation: using speech recognition and semantic analysis technology to complete examination and evaluation.
2. Personalized Learning Plan: collecting information about each individual medical student and formulating personalized learning strategies, to create unique and featured learning experiences.
3. Detecting Problems in Students' Learning: using AI to continuously track the learning process of students (knowledge structure, ability level, learning needs) efficiently over time and find the deficiencies existing in knowledge structures, capabilities, or learning demands.
4. Cultivating the Clinical Thinking Patterns: IBM's Watson Health employs natural language, hypothesis generation, and evidence-based learning capabilities to aid clinical decision-making, and to support medical students in acquiring clinical thinking patterns (Bin et al. 2019).
5. Artificial Intelligence Expert System: professional knowledge, disciplinary experience, or typical cases in related fields are integrated into a database and stored in a computer, so that it can simulate the decision-making and thinking process of human experts, and output the analysis and judgment of practical problems by calculating and reasoning about the input information (Fujun et al. 2020).

1.2 Evaluation of the Application of AI in Medical Education

Reviews of the effectiveness of AI's applications in medical education are varied. In general, at present, AI technology is on the ascendant, and almost all fields attempt to combine with it to accelerate their own iterative upgrades and achieve breakthroughs in the speed and effectiveness of the industries' development. Medical education, including the teaching of clinical theories and techniques in anesthesiology, is no exception. Most medical education institutions and experts maintain an open attitude toward the introduction of AI, while some of them are actively promoting the organic integration of medical education and AI technologies, which can alleviate the existing dilemma of manpower shortage and inefficient use of resources. However, some experts also note that the development of technology is not simply a multidisciplinary superposition, and although various problems and obstacles are inevitable in the initial stage, early identification of problems, constant adjustment, and pushing forward the new is the focus and direction of the efforts of those who are committed to using AI technology to promote medical teaching.

Li et al. evaluated the effectiveness of the application of artificial intelligence expert systems in teaching clinical anesthesia techniques through experiments, surveys, and analysis. Firstly, a total of 160 students were divided into control and experimental groups, with the control group being taught with the traditional anesthesia teaching model and the experimental group learning through the artificial intelligence expert system model. After 2 weeks of study, both groups were evaluated in terms of theoretical knowledge of anesthesia and anesthesia clinical operation. The assessment was scored by three experts. At the same time, a survey on students' satisfaction with the teaching model was conducted in the form of a questionnaire, which the students had to complete within 20 min and scored 100 points. The survey was conducted in five dimensions, including the overall evaluation of the course, clinical needs matching, knowledge accessibility, course format, and student participation (Fujun et al. 2020).

Statistical analysis was performed on the assessment results and satisfaction survey results. Epidata 3.0 software was used for double entry and quality control of the quantitative data of the participants' assessment scores and satisfaction questionnaires; SPSS 18.0 was used for statistical analysis of all quantitative data. The measurement data were expressed as mean ± standard deviation ($x \pm s$), and the assessment and satisfaction scores between the two groups were tested by independent samples *t*-test, and the difference

($P < 0.05$) was considered statistically significant (Fujun et al. 2020).

The analysis of results included two aspects: (1) Comparison of assessment results. The scores of anesthesia theoretical and practical knowledge in the experimental group were higher than those in the control group, with the former $t = 2.583$, $P = 0.019 < 0.05$, and the latter $t = 2.374$, $P = 0.020 < 0.05$, both with statistically significant differences; (2) Comparison of satisfaction scores. Same to the results of the participants' knowledge assessment, the satisfaction scores of the experimental group's teaching mode were higher than the control group in all five dimensions, $t = 10.377$, $P = 0.001 < 0.05$, and the differences were statistically significant (Fujun et al. 2020).

Indeed, the study of Li et al. had several limitations. First of all, the sample size of the study population was small (160 participants). Secondly, information on the AI expert system was not presented in sufficient detail and there was no discussion of its generalizability for replication in other institutions. For example, the actual level of need and skills for anesthesia operation techniques were not exactly the same in different hospitals, e.g., hospitals focusing on organ transplantation and plastic surgery may differ in their anesthesia skill needs, with the former focusing on patient vital sign monitoring and pain management during surgery, while the latter may more frequently encounter difficult airway situations. Whether the role of artificial intelligence expert systems for medical student training and anesthesia teaching was optimistically positive for this situation remains to be investigated.

Other experts also suggested that although there were already fruits of the combination of AI with anesthesia clinical skills training, the application of AI in medical teaching was still insufficient, partly because of the special nature of anesthesia teaching and partly because of the limitations of existing technologies. The former included a large amount of data, a long duration, the existence of individualized differences, and understaffed instructors. The latter included the fact that existing developments are often built on the achievements of existing AI technologies and their applications in teaching, making it difficult to acquire truly innovative developments; current applications aimed more at alleviating the imminent problem of staffing shortages than at standardizing the envisaged training assessment (qualitative analysis) and developing individualized training programs. It is hoped that an in-depth analysis of existing problems will provide ideas for future technological breakthroughs in related fields.

1. Compared with other disciplines, anesthesia clinical skills teaching data are characterized by a large amount of data, various influencing factors, and complicated core priorities, so it is difficult to analyze the data. At present, it is considered that students involved in anesthesia clinical skills training should master at least 28 major anesthesia operation skills. They are operation of mechanical ventilation, rapid induction of endotracheal intubation, simple breathing bag operation, anesthetic drug dose configuration and use, intravertebral anesthesia, epidural anesthesia, subarachnoid lumbar puncture, intraoperative management of intravenous anesthesia, intraoperative and postoperative resuscitation of critically ill patients, extrathoracic cardiac asynchronous direct current defibrillation, endotracheal implementation of endotracheal anesthesia, preoperative patient visits, manual ventilation using anesthesia machine techniques, mask oxygen administration and setting of mechanical ventilation, intraoperative observation of anesthesia management, common analgesic techniques, local infiltration anesthesia, controlled hypotensive techniques, observation and management of intraoperative adverse reactions, handling of the emergency night shift in anesthesiology, anesthesia record sheet and summary writing, reading reports or notes on professional foreign language literature, central venipuncture, pediatric tracheal intubation, peripheral nerve block anesthesia (cervical plexus, brachial plexus), central venous pressure monitoring technique, jaw-holding method (open airway and invasive arterial puncture technique). The key

points for teaching assessment and feedback on mastering these anesthesia skills are different, and each anesthesiology postgraduate student performs a large number of clinical skills every day, which means that a large amount of teaching data is generated. It is difficult to provide accurate, timely, and efficient feedback through manual analysis by the supervising instructors.
2. Unlike the "grouped and unified" clinical skills training of other disciplines, most of the daily clinical skills training of anesthesiology postgraduates is carried out in their own operating rooms facing different patients, and they often need to complete the anesthesia management of several surgical patients and handle multiple clinical skills in a short period of time every day, so the demand for supervising teaching is high. Whereas, it is difficult for supervisors to provide timely, continuous, and effective teaching evaluation and feedback.
3. In previous clinical skills training and evaluation, instructors often observed and provided feedback on students' skills based on previously designed forms, often ignoring individual differences among patients, and did not include clinical anesthesia-related medical data (including quality of intraoperative anesthesia management, adverse events, quality of postoperative recovery, length of hospital stay and ICU time, medical costs, patient satisfaction, and comfort), which are the ultimate reflection of the quality of anesthesia clinical skills training.
4. There is a serious shortage of instructors for clinical anesthesia skills training. At present, one anesthesiology instructor has to be in charge of several or even more than ten specialized students in major teaching hospitals, which makes it difficult to provide high-quality education. These problems are difficult to be solved by the current teaching mode, and better means of intervention are needed to further improve the quality of training. If we design and study the database of clinical skills training assessment based on AI and apply it to the clinical training of postgraduate students in anesthesiology, it will facilitate the solution of the above problems and alleviate the pressure of a serious shortage of clinical anesthesiology teaching faculty, which is expected to significantly improve the teaching quality.

1.3 Directions for Improvement of AI in Clinical Skills Training

The goal of anesthetic clinical skills training is to reduce the dependence of the training on instructors and to improve the quality of clinical training. To be specific, the expected results include automatically diagnosing and tracking the weaknesses and deficiencies of the clinical skills of postgraduate students, providing a realistic and effective assessment of each anesthesiology students' absorption of skills during training, customizing individualized clinical training plan, and effectively offering solutions to the common problems currently faced by major medical schools.

2 The Application of AI in Anesthesiology Clinical Skills Training and Assessment in Other Countries

Research in other countries intended to reveal the current state of how AI participating in and assisting medical education, including the promotion of instruction's assessment, and how both instructors and students viewing AI's participation. The results alluded to the requirement for familiarizing graduate clinical students with AI technologies so that they can better utilize AI to provide professional and efficient healthcare services to patients in their future medical practice. Also, machine learning can provide high-quality and usable feedback which is valuable for the creation of improvement plans for trainees.

Banerjee et al. conducted a study to investigate the use of AI in medical teaching in the UK. In their study, Banerjee et al. evaluated the impact of AI technology on clinical education and also made recommendations for the use of AI in training based on the evaluation results with the aim of maximizing the benefits of clinical AI while mitigating the potential negative effects and concerns of AI. They collected the evaluation of doctors in NHS postgraduate training centers in London, UK on the application of AI in medical education and clinical training through a questionnaire. After analysis in scientific ways, it was eventually found that more than half of the doctors thought that clinical AI had a positive effect on training, while most of them said that the application of AI-related technologies in clinical training was far from adequate. Trainees thought that the artificial intelligence-based decision support system can automatically be updated with the latest literature which provided them convenient access to the latest academic evidence that not only enriched their theoretical knowledge but also instructed and guided their clinical practice. On the other hand, part of the respondents opposed such a convenience because they were concerned about the deskilling impact of AI technologies (Banerjee et al. 2021).

As Banerjee et al. appealed that clinical education must change along with clinical practice development, their study threw the need for formal AI training in clinical curricula into sharp relief, responding to the strong need for it among physicians in training. The influence of AI on medical education took different routes, namely direct and indirect ones. The direct impact refers to the AI technology can improve the delivery of the training itself, while the indirect impact is to benefit education by streamlining workflows and freeing up more time for education and training. Although the majority of respondents in their survey (72%) had not yet encountered AI systems regularly in training and education, this is an area of active research, ranging from assisted radiology teaching to virtual reality for surgical skills development (Aeckersberg et al. 2019) and automated assessment of procedure performance (Winkler-Schwartz et al. 2019). Medical curricula should be reexamined to force these technologies to directly promote the delivery of clinical education.

They recommended that medical curriculum developers reflect a new set of AI-specific skills. Data entry and management, mathematics and statistics, communicating AI results to patients, and AI-specific ethics were useful to be included. Traditional medical training curricula were saturated with limited room for new contents; thus, hands-on training in "applied AI" would be appropriate to a large extent. In addition to an overview of common ML architectures, this should include balanced training in clinical AI interpretation such as data bias, overfitting, and the potential for impairment (Banerjee et al. 2021).

Another similar study surveying radiologists and radiology residents' opinions of applying AI to medical education was conducted in Croatia and a consistent conclusion was produced that education on AI should be part of medical students' curricula (Dumić-Čule et al. 2020).

Assessment models of residents' performance were also designed and tested. Neves et al. applied machine learning models to accelerate the evaluation of the quality of attending feedback on resident performance (Neves et al. 2021). They argued that high-quality and usable feedback could create improvement plans for trainees, but that current manual assessments of the quality of such feedback were time consuming and subjective, and therefore they suggested seeking machine learning to quickly distinguish the quality of attending feedback on resident performance. Using a preexisting database of 1925 manually reviewed feedback comments from four anesthesiology residency programs (Beth Israel Deaconess Medical Center, University of Rochester Medical Center, University of Kentucky College of Medicine, and University of California San Diego), the authors trained machine learning models to predict whether comments contained six pre-defined feedback characteristics (actionable, behavior-focused, detailed, negative feedback, professionalism/communication, and specific) and to predict utility scores for comments on a scale of 1–5. Reviews with ≥ 4 feedback features were categorized as high-quality reviews and reviews with ≥ 4 utility scores were categorized as highly useful; otherwise, reviews were considered as low-quality or low-utility reviews, respectively.

They employed the data science platform RapidMiner Studio (RapidMiner, Inc., Boston, MA) to train, validate, and score the performance of the model. The results showed that the accuracy of predicting models in the presence of feedback features ranged from 74.4% to 82.2%. Prediction accuracy for the utility category was 82.1%, sensitivity was 89.2%, and class accuracy for the low-utility prediction was 89.8%. The prediction accuracy for the quality category was 78.5%, the sensitivity was 86.1%, and the class accuracy for the low-quality prediction was 85.0%. A research assistant with no machine learning experience spent 15–20 h familiarizing with the software, creating the model, and reviewing the performance of the predictions. The program read the data, applied the model, and generated predictions within minutes. In comparison, a recent author spent 15 h manually organizing and scoring 200 reviews over a 2-week period. As a result, they gave conclusions about the potential of using machine learning to quickly assess attending physician feedback on resident performance. Using predictive models to quickly screen out low-quality and low-utility feedback can help programs improve the delivery of feedback, both globally and to individual faculty members (Neves et al. 2021).

Globally, skills training for medical interventions is transitioning from a time-based model to a competency-based model. Holden et al. introduced that in the old time-based model, trainees would practice interventions for a fixed period of time, at which time they would be considered competent and graduate, or they would be considered ineligible and have to undergo remedial training. In the new competency-based model, trainees practiced until they reached a predetermined benchmark of competency. This program allowed each trainee to reach competency precisely within the required practice time. The disadvantage of this approach, however, was that trainees' competencies need to be constantly monitored (Holden et al. 2019). Expert-based skill assessment methods included checklists, global rating scales, and delegated scoring. Although these methods provided reliable assessments, especially when used in combination, they are expert dependent. As the number of medical classes increased and the demand for expert time increased, widespread implementation of expert-based assessments was not feasible. Instead, skill assessments should be automated (Neves et al. 2021).

Automated skill assessments can be applied to many different interventions (e.g., laparoscopic surgery, open surgery, and needle insertion) and can use data from many sources (e.g., instrument tracking, video, surgeon status, and patient monitors) (Reiley et al. 2011; Vedula et al. 2017). Perhaps the most common approach to automated skill assessment is metric-based assessment. In this model, clinical experts specified which aspects of the intervention are relevant to operator skills. Subsequently, these can be implemented into a set of performance metrics: quantities that can be understood by trainees and clinicians and can be easily calculated from measurable data. From these performance metrics, overall skill levels can be derived using pattern recognition or machine learning methods (Neves et al. 2021).

Metric-based overall skill assessment was initially approached as an optimization problem in which each metric was considered a cost and the most skilled operator was the one who could best weigh and minimize the cost. Since then, pattern recognition methods have been used to achieve increased reliability in assessment. Chmarra et al. showed that linear discriminant analysis reliably distinguished between novices and intermediaries as well as experts in laparoscopic training tasks (Chmarra et al. 2010). Similarly, Allen et al. showed that support vector machines outperformed cost-based methods for skill classification in laparoscopic training tasks (Allen et al. 2010). Oropesa et al. also demonstrated that support vector machines outperformed linear discriminant analysis and adaptive neuro-fuzzy inference systems in laparoscopic training tasks (Oropesa et al. 2014). Ahmidi et al. used support vector machines to classify skills in septoplasty for several different types of performance metrics for skill classification (Ahmidi et al. 2015). Fard et al. compared support vector machines with K-nearest neighbors and logistic regression for identifying novices and experts in robotic suturing tasks on real patients (Fard et al. 2017). Kramer et al. suggested learning vector quantization and self-organizing maps for the evaluation of simulated vascular surgery (Kramer et al. 2016). Neural network-based approaches have seen some success (Uemura et al. 2018). Fuzzy pattern recognition methods have also gained some attention, including rule-based approaches and adaptive fuzzy inference systems (Neves et al. 2021).

In consultation with clinical experts, the authors suggested that metric-based skill assessment methods should meet two criteria in order to be useful in clinical settings: transparency and configurability. A machine learning method was considered transparent if the model was easy to interpret and the main elements of the method were easy to understand (Kotsiantis 2007; Chiticariu et al. 2015). A machine learning method was considered configurable if its parameters can be configured to improve performance based on domain knowledge provided by domain experts (a component of transparency according to Chiticariu et al. (2015)). In interventional skills assessment, transparency allowed both supervisors and trainees to understand why trainees received a particular score and to interpret their results as actionable strategies to improve performance. Configurability allows experts to adapt assessments to their particular training scenario or to emphasize specific skills (Neves et al. 2021).

3 Conclusion

Clinical artificial intelligence will impact medical education and clinical training. Artificial intelligence systems can be developed to not only classify participants based on surgical expertise but also guide trainees to a defined surgical standard. These systems will allow research to be conducted to further elaborate appropriate methods for the use of AI in the teaching of anesthesia operative skills. Training in practical procedures and clinical judgment may be simplified by the clinical AI systems, and educational opportunities for these skills should be guaranteed. Trained physicians have an overall positive view of the impact. Regardless of the future, a clear understanding of best practices in surgery, AI approaches, and education will be critical to the eventual successful application of AI technologies in clinical teaching.

References

Aeckersberg G, Gkremoutis A, Schmitz-Rixen T, Kaiser E. The relevance of low-fidelity virtual reality simulators compared with other learning methods in basic endovascular skills training. J Vasc Surg. 2019;69(1):227–35. https://doi.org/10.1016/j.jvs.2018.10.047.

Ahmidi N, Poddar P, Jones JD, Vedula SS, Ishii L, Hager GD, Ishii M. Automated objective surgical skill assessment in the operating room from unstructured tool motion in septoplasty. Int J Comput Assist Radiol Surg. 2015;10(6):981–91.

Allen B, Nistor V, Dutson E, Carman G, Lewis C, Faloutsos P. Support vector machines improve the accuracy of evaluation for the performance of laparoscopic training tasks. Surg Endosc. 2010;24(1):170–8.

Banerjee M, Chiew D, Patel KT, Johns I, Chappell D, Linton N, Cole GD, Francis DP, Szram J, Ross J, Zaman S. The impact of artificial intelligence on clinical education: perceptions of postgraduate trainee doctors in London (UK) and recommendations for trainers. BMC Med Educ. 2021;21(1):429. https://doi.org/10.1186/s12909-021-02870-x.

Bin Y, Yuwen C, Kunhua Z, et al. Application of artificial intelligence in clinical skill training and assessment of master of anesthesiology. Medical Education Research and Practice. 2019;29(3):421–5.

Chiticariu L, Li Y, Reiss F. Transparent machine learning for information extraction: state-of-the-art and the future. In: Conference on empirical methods in natural language processing; 2015. p. 4–6.

Chmarra MK, Klein S, de Winter JCF, Jansen F-WW, Dankelman J. Objective classification of residents based on their psychomotor laparoscopic skills. Surg Endosc Other Interv Tech. 2010;24(5):1031–9.

Dumić-Čule I, Orešković T, Brkljačić B, Kujundžić Tiljak M, Orešković S. The importance of introducing artificial intelligence to the medical curriculum – assessing practitioners' perspectives. Croat Med J. 2020;61(5):457–64. https://doi.org/10.3325/cmj.2020.61.457.

Fard MJ, Ameri S, Darin Ellis R, Chinnam RB, Pandya AK, Klein MD. Automated robot-assisted surgical skill evaluation: predictive analytics approach. Int J Med Robot Comput Assist Surg. 2017;14(1):e1850.

Fujun L, Qiuyan Y, Yue L, et al. Application and research of artificial intelligence expert system on teaching in anesthesiology. Chinese Hospital Management. 2020;40(8):73–5.

Holden MS, Xia S, Lia H, Keri Z, Bell C, Patterson L, Ungi T, Fichtinger G. Machine learning methods for automated technical skills assessment with instructional feedback in ultrasound-guided interventions. Int J Comput Assist Radiol Surg. 2019;14(11):1993–2003. https://doi.org/10.1007/s11548-019-01977-3. Epub 2019 Apr 20

Kotsiantis SB. Supervised machine learning: a review of classification techniques. Informatica. 2007;31:249–68.

Kramer BD, Losey DP, O'Malley MK, O'Malley MK. SOM and LVQ classification of endovascular surgeons using motion-based metrics. In: Merényi E, Mendenhall MJ, O'Driscoll P, editors. Advances in self-organizing maps and learning vector quantization: proceedings of the 11th international workshop WSOM 2016, Houston, Texas, USA, January 6–8, 2016, vol. 428. Cham: Springer; 2016. p. 227–37.

Neves SE, Chen MJ, Ku CM, Karan S, DiLorenzo AN, Schell RM, Lee DE, Diachun CAB, Jones SB, Mitchell JD. Using machine learning to evaluate attending feedback on resident performance. Anesth Analg. 2021;132(2):545–55. https://doi.org/10.1213/ANE.0000000000005265.

Oropesa I, Sánchez-González P, Chmarra MK, Lamata P, Pérez-Rodríguez R, Jansen FW, Dankelman J, Gómez EJ. Supervised classification of psychomotor competence in minimally invasive surgery based on instruments motion analysis. Surg Endosc Other Interv Tech. 2014;28(2):657–70.

Reiley CE, Lin HC, Yuh DD, Hager GD. Review of methods for objective surgical skill evaluation. Surg Endosc. 2011;25(2):356–66.

Uemura M, Tomikawa M, Miao T, Souzaki R, Ieiri S, Akahoshi T, Lefor AK, Hashizume M. Feasibility of an AI-based measure of the hand motions of expert and novice surgeons. Comput Math Methods Med. 2018;2018:9873273. https://doi.org/10.1155/2018/9873273.

Vedula SS, Ishii M, Hager GD. Objective assessment of surgical technical skill and competency in the operating room. Annu Rev Biomed Eng. 2017;19(1):301–25.

Winkler-Schwartz A, Bissonnette V, Mirchi N, Ponnudurai N, Yilmaz R, Ledwos N, Siyar S, Azarnoush H, Karlik B, del Maestro RF. Artificial intelligence in medical education: best practices using machine learning to assess surgical expertise in virtual reality simulation. J Surg Educ. 2019;76(6):1681–90. https://doi.org/10.1016/j.jsurg.2019.05.015.

Limitations and Ethical Implications of Artificial Intelligence

Bifa Fan

As artificial intelligence (AI) systems develop and mature in health care, they will be used in a wide range of clinical applications. Yet, it is not without its limitations. Currently, AI medicine is still hardly applicable in clinical settings because of its immaturity. It is highly reliant on human doctors and high-tech machines. It could only show the final result, without explanation and supportive details. Moreover, its dubious accuracy, complexity of usage, and other problems make medical institutions hesitate in the adoption of AI medicine. For the general public, it is critical to understand that using AI-based techniques will not necessarily result in classification or prediction that is superior to current methods. AI is a tool that must be deployed in the right situation to solve an appropriate problem.

With the gradual progress of AI medicine, it will surely bring impact to the traditional medical model, which in turn brings new social, economic, and legal problems. While constructing electronic medical records for patients for therapy, AI collects a large amount of data from one single patient. Patient privacy would be a topic worth discussing. Meanwhile, it remains uncertainty as to which party should bear legal liability for AI-produced results. Another issue is when AI takes over work in the medical field, there would be fewer job vacancies left for the human labor force. How to deal with the many problems brought by AI and ensure its safe and controlled development are issues that must be taken seriously and solved now.

1 Limitations

1.1 Reliance on Human Doctors and Expensive Equipment

AI is making strides in the field of medicine. However, AI is not yet fully independent in making diagnoses when truly in clinical settings. It needs to work in collaboration with medical staff. It also requires the integration of various complex devices and the building of a cloud platform to assist analysis of big medical data. For instance, the image acquisition of ultrasound AI needs to be done manually by physicians, and the physician's practice has a direct impact on AI diagnosis. Therefore, the application of ultrasound AI requires experienced physicians and intelligent diagnostic systems to work together in a regular and coordinated manner. Physician training on AI-assisted diagnostic technology should be conducted regularly to equip operators with qualified technical skills. In addition, the programmed diagnosis of the machine may create a gap between doctors and patients and weaken the multidisciplinary joint diagnosis of

B. Fan (✉)
Department of Pain Management, China-Japan Friendship Hospital, Beijing, China

M. Xia, H. Jiang (eds.), *Artificial Intelligence in Anesthesiology*,
https://doi.org/10.1007/978-981-99-5925-9_12

diseases. Therefore, to take advantage of AI in diagnosis, the synergy between machines and humans must be well done.

1.2 Black Box Results

One criticism of AI, and neural networks in particular, is that these approaches can lead to black box results, where an algorithm can provide a predicted outcome for a clinician or researcher but cannot reveal further information about the reason that such a prediction was made. Explainable AI is working to improve the transparency of algorithms. It targets on producing models that can more easily clarify their prediction, for example, by demonstrating features on which making predictions may depend, with the ultimate goal of increasing the transparency of algorithms and models, and thus strengthening human trust and understanding of its predictions. Some techniques in AI are easier to explain than others. For example, decision trees allow for great transparency since each decision node can be reviewed and evaluated, whereas deep learning is currently assessed by induction. In other words, each node in a deep learning model may not be able to clearly explain why certain predictions are made; but the model can present relevant features or examples from its training data of skeletal X-rays that can somehow explain why a particular prediction was made about the bone age of a patient (Lee et al. 2017). Apart from concerns over transparency and trust in models, AI also performs well in demonstrating correlations or in identifying patterns, but it cannot yet determine causal relationships, or at least not to a degree that satisfies the requirements of clinical implementation. With more researches exploring the field, clinicians must critically review new research findings and product announcements. At the same time, medical education and training should incorporate a literacy component to the concept of AI.

For anesthesiologists, understanding the internal mechanisms of machine learning models is very difficult. Neural networks and machine learning can process large amounts of data and generate extremely complex models, but it is difficult for humans to understand or interpret the machine output. Multiple operations in computer algorithms can lead to an obvious black box phenomenon: machine learning data analysis is done through complex functions or models that are difficult for humans to understand the output. For example, in a neural network, a single neuron receives input signals from multiple neurons, and after weighting and summing these signals, the summed signals are passed to the subsequently connected neurons, and so on, with the subsequent neurons again receiving input signals from the previous layer of neurons. If the above steps are repeated, multiple layers of operations are created between the input and output ports. The output of the computer depends on the machine learning model and algorithm, and it is difficult for the anesthesiologist to determine whether there are arithmetic errors inside its "black box." Therefore, the opaqueness and unexplainability of the operation mode of the machine learning model will greatly limit its application. More explainable anticipation and more supported result is necessary before clinicians can reassuringly embrace AI as a fundamental tool.

1.3 Difficulty in Application

Medicine is a science with a very low tolerance for error, and the accuracy of AI's auxiliary diagnostic results could not be higher. Only with high accuracy and specificity can its value in clinical applications be better utilized. The database and the construction of algorithmic models are important conditions that affect the diagnostic accuracy of AI medicine. For example, the application of ultrasound AI requires access to high-quality ultrasound image data and active participation of high-level specialist physicians, and deep learning through accurate data annotation and reasonable model design. AI algorithms need to overcome the bias of different data and be jointly optimized by experienced clinicians and algorithm engineers. Data, algorithms, and computing power are the basic three elements of AI. Among them, high-precision training data is the basis for applying AI. The data used for training should not only pursue "quantity," but also "quality." At present, the data source of AI is limited to a single center or a multi-center study in a local area, and the data collection equipment is not uniform, which will affect the accuracy and standardization of the data, leading to wrong output results and affecting the stability and safety of AI.

Moreover, AI algorithms are rather vulnerable to bias in data. Apart from the basic research biases that clinicians have learned such as sampling and blinding, both implicit and explicit bias in the healthcare system that can impact the large-scale data that is or will be used to train AI should also be considered. Eligibility of specific patient populations for clinical trials, implicit biases in treatment decisions in real-world care, and other forms of bias can profoundly influence the types of predictions that AI may make and clinical decisions (Murthy et al. 2004; Schulman et al. 1999). Char et al. (2018) gave the example of withdrawal of treatments from patients with traumatic brain injury. AI may analyze data from a neuro-ICU and interpret patterns of death following traumatic brain injury as an inevitable consequence of the injury rather than as a secondary cause of clinical decisions to withdraw life support. Consequently, it is imperative that practicing clinicians partner or engage in a dialogue with data scientists to guarantee the appropriate interpretation of data analyses.

2 Ethical Implications

2.1 Privacy Issues

In addition to the difficulty of data collection and data analysis, researchers also face another challenge—data protection. With the development of the Internet, the risk of data loss or even patient privacy exposure due to hacking into the database will further increase. Privacy leakage has become one of the most prominent factors limiting the development of AI. Currently, China lacks relevant laws and regulations to regulate the privacy protection of health data. Therefore, when applying AI, not only do researchers need to take strong security measures to prevent health data leakage and hackers' intrusion or control of the database, but also the government and relevant regulatory authorities need to formulate perfect laws, regulations, and monitoring systems to regulate the reasonable use of data.

2.2 Legal Liabilities

The rapid development of AI technology brings new risks and challenges to the access and regulation of its products. Ultrasound AI products are innovative R&D products and the current system in terms of technical management norms, technical access, and application fees is lacking and requires continuous improvement in management. China has some policies to respond to the arrival of AI. In 2017, the former National Health and Family Planning Commission formulated the Management Specification for AI-assisted Diagnostic Technology and the Quality Control Index for Clinical Application of AI-assisted Diagnostic Technology, which set the basic requirements for medical institutions and medical personnel to carry out AI-assisted diagnosis. In 2018, the China Ultrasound Medical AI (USAI) Code of Conduct—Beijing Declaration was released to promote the development and application of AI in ultrasound medicine and to promote the deep integration and healthy development of ultrasound and AI development. However, there is not yet a new department dedicated to the review of digital healthcare and AI technologies, while the United States has started to set up a relevant department to look into the future development of AI and its broad impact on society (Jiang et al. 2018). In the next step, the field of medicine should establish a scientific regulatory system for AI, improve the laws and regulations for ultrasound AI applications, further improve the scheme for assessing the stability and accuracy of AI, and overcome the difficulty of defining medical liability for AI.

2.3 Unemployment

Many scholars are worried that while bringing convenience for human beings by freeing people of repetitive work, the development of AI would threaten low-skilled workers as they would take their job opportunities. Smith and Anderson (2014), Pajarinen et al. (2015), Frey and Osborne (2017) have shown that a significant portion of future jobs will be replaced by machines, especially programmed and standardized jobs; Goddard et al. (2021) found through their studies that the use of AI technologies will not only replace the vast majority of routine jobs, but even threaten some non-routine jobs as well. Wang et al. (2017) argued that AI technology develops faster and covers a wider area, and a large number of companies save the use of labor at a higher rate in order to create greater benefits, so much so that it exceeds the rate of job creation, which can trigger unemployment.

For sure, the field of AI would open a gate of new job vacancies as machines require operative workers and maintenance workers. Yet it remains a question if jobs created by AI could outnumber the ones taken by it.

Now, AI in medicine is still in the primary stage and does not have the function of communication. Therefore, AI is currently more applied in areas like image recognition-assisted analysis that do not require in-depth communication with patients, and the application of other areas still needs the continued improvement of AI technology. In the future, AI will play an increasingly important role in the medical field, promoting the development of medicine, and reshaping the medical industry. It is believed that AI will bring profound changes to future medical technology and is a powerful driving force for future medical innovation and reform. And it is crucial that the general public is well prepared for that. While safely conducting the gradual implementation of AI techniques in medicine, care should also be taken to protect human rights. Researchers need to make efforts in enhancing the accuracy and applicability of AI while making the least intrusion into patients' privacy. The government should perfect relative laws and regulations, specifying legal liabilities, while ensuring job opportunities for medical workers and protecting data privacy for patients. Medical institutions should provide thorough and profound training for medical employees, including the proper usage, the underlying logic, and interpretation of the results of a particular AI method. All forces should be combined together while smoothly improving AI's performance in the medical field.

3 Summary

Like all other new techniques, AI has its issues in its application and integration into different fields, and in the medical field, these issues can be generally divided into two groups, namely its limitations and ethical problems. For limitations, AI in the medical field still has the reliance on human operators, which hinders the realization of higher efficiency; AI also produces results that are usually considered to be in the "black box" and lack transparency; at the same time, AI is difficult to apply in the medical field, which again poses a high requirement to its operators. For ethical problems, AI functions on the basis of a great load of data, which brings potential problems related to privacy and legal liabilities; in addition, the integration of AI means fewer job vacancies for human resources, which will in the end lead to unemployment. As simply summarized in this chapter, AI is never a flawless technique, therefore, it should not be abused blindly. The introduction of new technology first obliges human beings to accept it, then corresponding measures to facilitate its integration, for example, related laws and regulations, which is a big subject left for those who are studying AI to deal with.

References

Char DS, Shah NH, Magnus D. Implementing machine learning in health care – addressing ethical challenges. N Engl J Med. 2018;378:981–3.

Frey CB, Osborne M. The future of employment. Technol Forecast Soc Change. 2017;114:254–80.

Goddard MA, Davies ZG, Guenat S. A global horizon scan of the future impacts of robotics and autonomous systems on urban ecosystems. Nat Ecol Evol. 2021;5(2):219–30.

Jiang L-Y, Wang X-J, Jin C-L. Application and admittance of artificial intelligence in health service industry. Chin J Health Policy. 2018;11(11):78–82.

Lee H, Tajmir S, Lee J, Zissen M, Yeshiwas BA, Alkasab TK, Choy G, Do S. Fully automated deep learning system for bone age assessment. J Digit Imaging. 2017;30:427–41.

Murthy VH, Krumholz HM, Gross CP. Participation in cancer clinical trials: race-, sex-, and age based disparities. JAMA. 2004;291:2720–6.

Pajarinen M, Rouvinen P, Ekeland A. Computerization and the future of jobs in Norway [EB/OL]. The Research Institute of the Finnish Economy; 2015.

Schulman KA, Berlin JA, Harless W, Kerner JF, Sistrunk S, Gersh BJ, Dubé R, Taleghani CK, Burke JE, Williams S, Eisenberg JM, Escarce JJ. The effect of race and sex on physicians' recommendations for cardiac catheterization. N Engl J Med. 1999;340:618–26.

Smith A, Anderson J. AI, robotics, and the future of jobs. Pew Res Cent. 2014;6:51–8.

Wang J, Zhang Y-Z, Zhang Y-B, Hong Q-L. Mechanisms and countermeasures of new technological advances such as artificial intelligence affecting employment. Macroeconomics. 2017;10:169–81.

GPSR Compliance

The European Union's (EU) General Product Safety Regulation (GPSR) is a set of rules that requires consumer products to be safe and our obligations to ensure this.

If you have any concerns about our products, you can contact us on ProductSafety@springernature.com

In case Publisher is established outside the EU, the EU authorized representative is:

Springer Nature Customer Service Center GmbH
Europaplatz 3
69115 Heidelberg, Germany

Batch number: 10745899

Printed by Printforce, the Netherlands